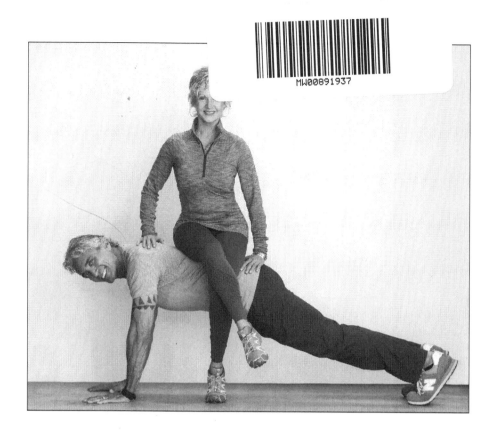

STACKING

Your Skeletal Blueprint for Posture

BY DEBBIE AND NORMAN COMPTON

ISBN: 978-1547247882

Editor: Michael McKnight

TABLE OF CONTENTS

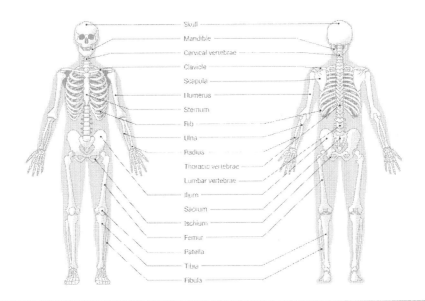

Skull
Mandible
Cervical vertebrae
Clavicle
Scapula
Humerus
Sternum
Rib
Ulna
Radius
Thoracic vertebrae
Lumbar vertebrae
Ilium
Sacrum
Ischium
Femur
Patella
Tibia
Fibula

The Skeletal System
Human Body Systems

INTRODUCTION

WHEN IT COMES TO KNOWLEDGE of the human musculoskeletal system, my husband Norm and I have been around the block. Through all of our personal challenges, and after nearly four decades of helping ourselves and others recover from injuries or other physical stresses brought on by poor postural habits, one fact emerges above all others. Achieving strength and balance, or successfully completing an injury rehabilitation program, are only temporary solutions if attention to one's posture, starting from the foundation, has not been part of the process.

Centuries of healers, researchers and doctors have written about the human body's amazing ability to heal and realign itself. Unlike other animals, our intelligence allows us to see an injury for what it is and address it, instead of only knowing it as an annoying ache or a bloody patch of fur. This book will include both old news and new science, but like our skeletons, if our writing isn't structured properly there will be imbalance and confusion. We have strived to make Stacking as clear as possible.

WHO ARE WE?

Norman and I have been together almost 40 years, but our young lives were from two different worlds. Norm, who is 62 as of this writing, was born and raised in Hawaii and was a well-rounded competitive athlete at a young age in the sports of football, baseball, rugby, soccer, and wrestling, and the less traditional pursuits of judo, swimming, surfing, outrigger canoe racing, and cliff diving. His name sounds haole (white) but Norm is "island" to his core, the proud son of a decorated (and Anglo) WWII vet and the Polynesian beauty he fell in love with.

In the mid 70s Norm joined the running craze and ran eleven marathons between 1978 and 1990. In 1983 he started doing stunt work on Magnum P.I., which led to a 27-year career as a Hollywood stuntman. At the age of 47, he became Dwayne "The Rock" Johnson's stunt double in the movie "Scorpion King."

I, on the other hand, grew up all over the Midwest. My father accumulated oil drilling rigs that kept our family moving from oil town to oil town in practically every state west of the Mississippi. Despite our nomadic ways, my parents managed to get me started in dance classes at five years old. That led to me performing with a company in ballet, jazz, and contemporary dance. In college at Oklahoma State University, I continued my dance education and was also a member of the Pom and Dance squads. Living in a variety of states throughout my youth brought proficiency in snow skiing and water skiing. I grew up hiking the Rockies. When I finished college, my older brother, a Marine fighter pilot, thought I deserved a celebratory trip and invited me to the Marine Officers Ball in a state I'd never been to: Hawaii. I went for the summer with a girlfriend and fell in love with island life. Two weeks before I was scheduled to leave, I met Norman. My friend went home. I stayed.

My physically active personality meshed with that of my new boy-friend. I joined Norm on four of his marathons, creating memories and stories that I'll share in the pages ahead. Norm also introduced this previously landlocked girl to the wonderful world of ocean sports, where I wasn't always graceful, but was always willing.

We were married in 1979. Within a year, Norm's job as one of Hawaii's more celebrated showroom entertainers took us to the island of Maui. With its beautiful ocean breezes and sunny skies, Maui would add something new to our already active lives. On Oahu, I had learned the art of distance running with Norm, but in Lahaina, for the first time, I experienced weight training. The year was 1980.

THE BIG THREE

While walking to town one day, we noticed that an old sugarcane cannery was being used as a gym. It definitely wasn't the type of gym one would envision by today's standards, but, simple as it was, it gave me my foundation. The benches were unpadded wood. A mishmash of rusty plates and dumbbells lay scattered beneath a roof of corru-gated steel. But you'll never catch me speaking ill of that place. We were in paradise, where nature rules all. This modest setting is where Norm taught me the Big Three—football's classic weightlifting pro-gram: bench press, power clean, squat. I didn't know it then, but these three movements would provide the foundation for a lifetime of body awareness.

In the beginning, however, I was sore! Still, I went to our rustic gym with Norm every day and did squats, power cleans, and bench. We shared what we were doing with the few people who asked us, but I recall one day in particular when we met a guy from the east coast who demonstrated a leg exercise we hadn't seen before. Instantly, we knew it would be long-term part of our training. This mainlander called them "lunges." Norm and I still do them daily, some 36 years later...

As fascinated 20-somethings, we tinkered and studied, and soon added side lunges and reverse lunges. We brought it all back to Oahu with us. Our desire for continued education—on the hows and whys of body mechanics—grew like the islands' wildflowers. We could feel the science and growth of this industry taking a positive turn.

When we were given the opportunity to train alongside the football team at the University of Hawaii (in what was known then as Klum Gym), Norm blended in easily. I, however, was intimidated and excited at the same time. All the equipment seemed so modern compared to the corrugated gym with unpadded wooden benches we had on Maui. Norm told me that my eagerness to learn and all that foundation work I learned in Lahina had these athletes' and coaches' encouraging me and led them to accept me as part of their Ohana (family). An entirely new world was revealing itself to me, and in the most beautiful setting imaginable.

Our commitment to the exploration of athletic possibilities brought people into our lives who were battling injury. Through our work with them, we began creating our own definition of health. This was the era of "no pain, no gain." Norm and I were fully entrenched in that scene, but we sensed that that mindset didn't fit what we were pursuing. We still value the sensations of burning lungs and legs, but our approach holds that there are enough things in life that are out of our control. Our health wasn't going to be one of them. On Oahu years ago, we began seeking a more nurturing, more respectful way to treat our bodies. A do-it-yourself counterbalance to the rigors that athletic competition puts us through.

With Norm's encouragement, I called on my dance background and began teaching aerobics classes starting on the lanai of the Canoe House at the Ilikai Hotel. It was a big step in that both of our jobs now exposed us to people from around the world. This led organically to requests for personal training, which was a new concept in Hawaii in the early 80s. When my aerobics clients asked for something new, like weight training, I'd reply: "Do you know the Big Three?" They most assuredly did not!

LIVING AND LEARNING

Each of these new relationships in some way reconfirmed our belief in building a foundation, building balance before building strength. The 80s and early 90s were a whirlwind of trial and (sometimes painful) error, of experience, and of research. To this day, we attend every relevant conference we can get to.

Norm and I, with what feels like a lifetime in this industry, have developed a menu of simple "assessments" that are geared toward finding solutions to pain and dysfunctional movement patterns. We look past traditional injury "rehab," which focuses only on the injured bones or hinges, and instead assess the entire musculoskeletal machine—including postural components that don't seem to play a role in a given injury (but secretly do). Smart injury rehab is a worthwhile pursuit, a necessary one, but finding the breakdown that caused the pain is our specialty. Once it's found, we believe in addressing the breakdown with two of nature's most potent medicines: alignment and movement.

My large-group aerobics classes were soon replaced by one-on-one sessions with athletes who had sport-specific injuries. Actors, models and other celebrities waded into our lives seeking a specific "look." Repeatedly we were told that, in addition to helping them work toward their goals, we were also helping them relieve unrelated imbalances. This was all done in a grass-roots manner in Hawaii. When we moved to California, we became certified in the field and I began working as a personal trainer full time.

I started in Redondo Beach, at Golds Gym. Eventually we moved to Hermosa Beach and I began working alongside one of the best strength and conditioning coaches in the world, Jeremy "Troll" Subin, owner of the renowned Yard Training Center. In addition to my work with post-partum mothers, weekend warriors, and injured athletes, I also developed a reputation for helping people with special needs. In the 27 years in the health industry in California there have been clients with issues ranging from obesity, to scoliosis, to Parkinson's disease, as well as those dealing with structural irregularities like hip abnormalities or webbed toes. And then there's Norm, who years ago labeled himself my "science project" in light of his often grueling 27-year career as a stuntman and actor in the movies. The injuries he incurred at work turned out to be far more unique than his sports injuries. Nearly four decades after we walked like wide-eyed kids into that rusty old gym on Maui, we are still learning,

In a way, this book represents the culmination of all those years. Just as we did in the 80s, each person we work with today is still assessed first as to the quality of his or her Stack, starting with the condition of the feet. We believe in training that progresses "from the bones out," as opposed to "from the muscles in."

On occasion, Norm or I have been the ones in need of an assessment. Considering our active jobs and lifestyles, sometimes we were the ones who needed to recover from injury as efficiently and thoroughly as possible. Norm has broken his collarbone at work, torn knee ligaments (during a stunt that required him to tumble down a flight of metal stairs) and broken his heel. In a split second, he tore the bicep and rotator cuff on both shoulders by simultaneously clotheslining two guys off their horses in "Scorpion King." Then there are his 11 completed marathons, and his old rugby and football injuries.

Our passion for new knowledge and research increases every year, and with every new ache or twinge we feel ourselves. Our focus on continuing education has allowed us to stay in touch with the constantly changing science within exercise and sport. Below is a condensed list of certifications I hold:

» MEDICAL EXERCISE SPECIALIST - trained to bring individuals back into balance after rehabilitation of an isolated injury, surgery, or structural imbalance.

» AMERICAN COUNCIL ON EXERCISE - HEALTH COACH - Among other benefits, this education provides connection with the medical community in the fields of Exercise Science, Nutritional Science, and Behavioral Science.

» POWER WALKING MASTER INSTRUCTOR, REEBOK UNIVERSITY - These instructors impart safety, proper technique, and scientific research pertaining to cardiovascular exercise.

» CERTIFIED FITNESS COACHING SPECIALIST - I am trained to create personalized program designs for individual clients' needs and goals.

» AMERICAN COUNCIL ON EXERCISE - A.C.E. certifies personal trainers.

The human body is an amazing creation. Our lifestyle either supports our ingenious physical machine, or challenges it. We all have different issues to address, but developing a strong skeletal "Stack" and learning to keep our bones in their pockets is a worthwhile start to any exercise program. Our contribution to this fascinating field is in your hands, *Stacking: Your Skeletal Blueprint for Posture.*

DEBBIE COMPTON
Redondo Beach, Calif.,
May 2017

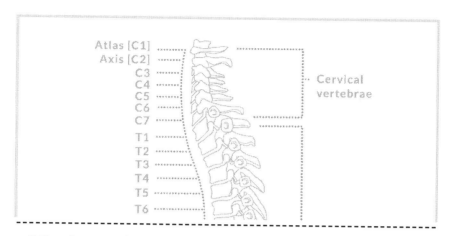

"The doctor of the future will give no medicine, but will interest his patients in the care of the human frame, in diet, and in the cause and prevention of disease."

- THOMAS EDISON

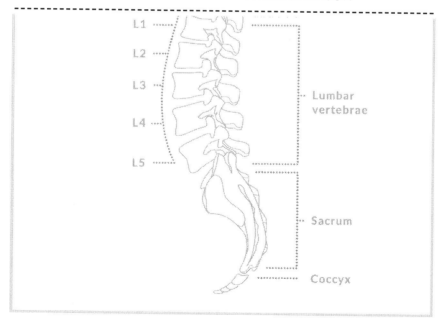

CHAPTER 1
Stacking

stacking (*noun*) — to build an orderly pile.

IMAGINE BEING PRESENTED WITH A PILE of 206 human bones, big and small, heaped haphazardly on the floor and being told to pile those bones in the correct alignment and sequence, starting with the feet and working up, until you have finished the skull and are looking at a complete human skeleton. One of your first questions (After, *Why am I doing this again?*) might be: *What is going to hold it all together? Glue? Some sort of scaffolding to hold everything in place while I continue to build upward?*

The task described above is what this book is all about. Our goal is to help you build the most stable, most functional skeleton possible, using your ligaments and tendons as the "glue," and your vast network of muscles as the scaffolding. As with any construction project, gravity will be our opponent. We can only complete our mission if the connections inside our skeletons are healthy, strong, and assembled just so.

We will want your completed skeleton to *move*, of course, and we'll also want it to remain undamaged, despite outside influences. So as we build we'll ask some of our muscles to act as mobilizers and others to act as stabilizers. Each section of this skeleton that we finish together will determine the health and durability of the sections surrounding it, so let's make sure that each bone we add to our stack rests in its best position, in its designated "pocket." Without these pockets, the forces of age and everyday wear-and-tear will topple what we have built. The structures above this weak link will be compromised, too.

A healthy, functioning knee that is positioned in a strong pocket, for example, must by definition be preceded by the construction of a stable foot, a stable ankle, a stable lower leg. If these lower sections of our stack are built haphazardly, or are allowed to fall into disrepair, the knee will suffer. (Followed by the hip. Then the spine. And so on.)

JOINT INTEGRITY

The concept of "joint integrity" is not just for competitive athletes. It's for everyone. Our daily lives present us with stairs, puddles, curbs, gravel—an accidental shove on the commuter train—all kinds of obstacles. Life often asks us to carry multiple grocery bags and children through this unpredictable world. It makes sense, then, to educate ourselves on how our bones and joints interact with each other—and with gravity—before we take on life's challenging errands.

Think of this book as an instruction manual that you are handed moments after you're ordered to arrange that messy pile of bones into a stack. The good news is that the glue and scaffolding are included (and free!).

Good health is a puzzle with many diverse pieces. Every cell in our bodies is somehow linked to every other cell. (We won't be discussing nutrition in this book other than to state that creating and maintaining a healthy "stack" requires a balanced diet rich in the six basic fuels—water, protein, carbohydrates, fat, vitamins, and minerals.)

Every physical activity can create imbalances. This is particularly true with work or sport activities performed at high repetitions, and even more so if these movements are not balanced with supportive exercises to counteract all those identical reps. It can take years for compensations to surface, but they almost always do. Many of this book's readers cracked open these pages for this exact reason: an injury brought on by repetitive activity. There are also plenty of people who have undergone joint replacement not due to overuse, but *underuse.* In these cases, supportive muscles have been neglected and are unable to perform their important jobs. Soon afterward, gravity takes over and creates chaos. Never underestimate gravity. We're no physicists, but we're pretty sure that gravity hasn't let up for a single second since shortly after earth was created.

This book aspires to help readers begin a communication with their bodies that will prevent imbalances and injuries. No one can force you to care about your body or the way it functions; our goal is simply to encourage a new respect for what most of the world's religions agree is "our temple." There are few more profound feelings than achieving deep knowledge and mastery of one's own physical being.

Our education starts with the skeletal system and the deep layer of underappreciated muscles and connectors that control it. We believe that the best way to improve posture is "from the bones out." Some of our most important muscles and connective tissues can't be seen in a mirror. These muscles—the ones closest to our bones—provide the strongest scaffolding for our stack. They guard against crumbling sections and slippages.

If you're recovering from a significant injury, a rehab plan that ignores your stack will provide a less than complete recovery. Organizing your posture from the ground up—and from the bones out—*has* to be part of the plan. It should also include re-training your healed area to interact with the uninjured structures above and below it. Ignoring these details almost always results in overcompensation, and – *POP!* – another injury.

JUDGE NOT

The process of communicating with and controlling our bodies starts when we define our postural foundation and begin constructing our stack.

Don't be fooled by appearances. Over the years we have worked with individuals who were born with webbed toes or fingers. One man in particular had webbing between the last three toes of his left foot. His whole life he had perceived this as a weakness, when in truth, his feet were structurally identical to our feet, or any other healthy person's feet. He spent his whole life compensating for a perfectly healthy foot. When he finally started a strength program at age 54, he learned that his chronically bad back was a by-product of this unnecessary psychological compensation.

Starting his assessment, as with every client, with his feet, we found over-dominant muscles that had taken over for muscles he'd ignored because they seemed weak. These ignored muscles had atrophied drastically. We also found a mixture of over-tight and over-stretched muscles and connectors, and a chronically weak ankle that we felt could be made strong again. The medial (inside) portion of his left knee was compromised. He had dangerously weak adductors (inner thigh muscles). His postural stack was a heap of rubble. The main result of this chaos? Excruciating lower back pain.

We're all different in terms of pain threshold – the point at which the body says, "No more." Without proper stacking, this threshold becomes thinner, more acute. As we build our stack, chapter by chapter, bone by bone, the keys to neutralizing lower back pain will become clearer. As with most postural ailments, it usually begins with the feet. We will bang this drum often: *developing an awareness of the feet is a step that cannot be skipped*. It's also easier said than done, especially as we age.

A quick, related story:

Many years ago, shortly after Norm invited me to join him on his long-distance runs, he stopped and pointed out that my feet rotated outward when I ran. He couldn't explain it at the time, but instinct told him that this was not good. Ballet, a constant in my life since I was a girl, had reinforced in me the idea that toes-out is good and toes-forward is bad. After Norm's intervention, I became much more aware of what my feet were doing. I still am. Considering the miles of running that lay ahead of me back then, if Norm hadn't offered his advice that day, my knees, hips, and spine would be a hot mess right now.

I trained myself to return my feet "to neutral." (More about this later.) Those who spend time around us hear us say often: "If you're strong in neutral, you're strong everywhere." Align your body the way it's supposed to be aligned. Keep your bones in their "pockets," starting with the feet. A building will not stand for long if its foundation is crooked.

Many of us are wired to believe that if we feel discomfort during exercise, the solution is *more work*. Can you imagine how many millions of injuries this has caused over the years? The inverse reaction – which is also harmful – is to stop exercising altogether. Countless worthwhile fitness programs have met their premature end this way. The answer is not more work, or less work, but *correct work*. Allowing your miraculous stack of 206 bones to move the way it's designed to move.

And it all begins—here's that drumbeat again—with the feet, arguably the most crucial and most ignored parts of our musculoskeletal systems. You're tired of hearing about them already, but remember: don't judge based on appearance. Give your feet their due. In almost every physical endeavor, in almost every competitive sport, which body part makes contact with the ground most often? *The feet*. (Whatever comes next is in a very distant second.) So let's start by building our stack there, where the rubber meets the road. And remember:

When you're strong in neutral you're strong everywhere.

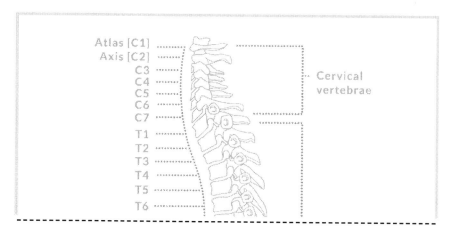

"Unless you change how you are, you will always have what you've got."

- JIM ROBIN

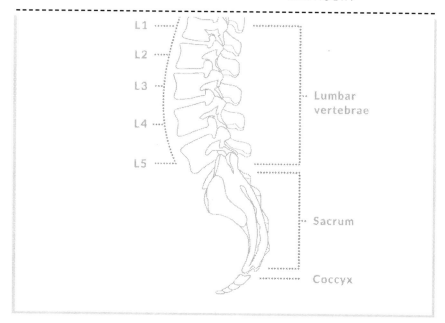

CHAPTER 2
The Triangle

OUR FEET WERE BUILT to support the weight of our bodies and to provide a stable platform when our bodies are in motion. The human foot has 26 bones and more than 100 muscles, ligaments, and tendons. Becoming aware of what the feet are doing at any given time will determine the health of the joints *above* the feet, such as the ankle, knee, and hip. The foundation provided by our feet is irreplaceable, whether you're a child learning to walk or an elite athlete recovering from knee surgery. Our first focus will be the four layers of muscle on the bottom of the foot.

Earlier I mentioned Norman's career as a stuntman. We had no idea that his career would provide not just paychecks, but an education for us in the body's resilience—its miraculous ability to heal and recover. Here's a stuntman story that involves the foot:

The movie was *Speed II*. The location was a luxury cruise ship. Norm was one of the stuntmen positioned in the lifeboats. They were portraying passengers, and when the ropes snapped their job was to plummet ten feet and crash into the ocean while standing in the boat.

Well, Norm's heel hit a metal rib in the boat's belly, fracturing his heel bone. Only an extreme impact can break this thick, solid bone—the calcaneus—and apparently a ten-foot drop onto a steel rod (which was on top of an unforgiving ocean) did the trick. The aftermath, in Norm's case, included pain that brought him to tears. To make a long story short, the show had to go on, so Norm endured several more painful weeks of work before he was able to get the broken heel addressed.

We were advised to start aggressive physical therapy, which we did. After several months, though, no healing had taken place. It became obvious that surgery was the only solution, but due to the tardiness of this decision his plantar fascia connector had thickened and a knot of scar tissue had formed. Even after this scar tissue was removed and the plantar fascia was partially snipped from its insertion point at the bone, Norm's gauntlet wasn't over. After months of developing an adjusted walk, we noticed that the upper calf muscle on the back of his knee had completely atrophied ... *on his uninjured leg*.

The point is: every muscle, ligament, and tendon has its own job – some do several jobs at once – and when a few of them aren't working properly (as with Norm's compromised plantar fascia), a domino trail of muscles, ligaments, and tendons are affected, even on the opposite leg. When normal muscle activity is disrupted, the surrounding structures compensate. It's a rule as constant as gravity.

By focusing on the long muscles of the feet, we forced Norm's atrophied calf muscle to contract. It took a lot of hard work on Norm's part, and it brought the added benefit of teaching him to *feel* the bottom of his feet, teaching him to find balance there, to distribute weight evenly among the three points of his "triangle." (See below.) Norm's crippling injury taught him how to begin building his stack.

(A quick aside: when Norm tells this story he always follows it with the tale of his friend, 70-year-old stuntwoman May Boss, who worked in the lifeboat with him on that shoot. Norm thought that the production team might take it easy on Mae in light of her advanced age. "She not only fell the 10 feet," Norm recalls, "she stuck the landing like a pro. *In high heels!*")

FINDING YOUR TRIANGLE

When assessing someone else's "stack," Norman and I always start at the bottom—the soles of the feet—and work our way up. Try this:

Sit in a firm chair with your knees and hips at 90 degrees, wearing no shoes. The triangle you're looking for is formed by the line of five joints where your toes begin—often called the balls of the feet—and two imaginary lines that connect this line to your heel. Using the muscles of the feet, press into the ground at the big toe joint (the largest ball of your foot), slowly moving one toe at a time to the smallest ball of your foot. We call this the "Toe Joint Line" or "Top of The Triangle." Now visualize the base of the heel bone, the point where it meets the ground. Place even pressure at the center of this point. With these two quick explorations, you have found your Triangle.

If your search comes up empty at first, don't be discouraged. Weak, tight muscles, and compromised nerves can make anyone's Triangle difficult to locate. Stay with it. By practicing these pressures into the ground, you are developing and strengthening the foot, and gaining a more balanced foundation.

It's easier to feel our Triangles when we're seated and barefoot, but you can also exercise them while standing in line at the bank or the grocery store. Remind yourself to distribute weight evenly on those three points. The higher structures in your "stack"—your hips and spine, to name two—will reap the benefits of the progress you make at ground level.

Learning to stretch the muscles on the bottom of the foot is another important step. Give this a shot:

In the same, seated position, simultaneously lift all five toes while keeping your Triangle planted. Hold for twenty seconds or so. Next, relax your toes and rise onto the toe joint line ("balls of your feet"), maintaining even distribution of your weight on all five joints and keeping the toes relaxed. Now stand up. Try these two movements in the standing position. For the standing heel raise, you can rest your hands on a stable surface to allow greater focus on the feet muscles. Avoid putting weight on the toes themselves—we call this "going past the joint line"—because this places undue stress on the connective tissue there. Our goal is to prevent pain, not create it.

Each of our five toes has its own job. These individual responsibilities will be strengthened each time we work on the Triangle. Think of your toes as extensions of your foot that provide you with balance during movement. They're small, but our toes are incredibly sturdy stabilizers. Here are six steps to making them even stronger.

STEP 1: From a seated position, "put your feet up" on an ottoman or chair. Working one foot at a time:

STEP 2: Point your toes like a ballerina, from the ankle downward. Feel the squeeze in your arch.

STEP 3: Now, pull your toes back toward your body *from the joint line* (balls of the feet), while maintaining your "toes pointed" position everywhere else (extended foot at the ankle).

STEP 4: Now flex your *entire foot* back toward your body, while keeping your toes in the raised/flexed position described in Step 3.

STEP 5: Keep your ankle flexed, but allow the toes to relax. You can perform these five valuable steps anytime, anywhere. When you've completed them on both feet, perform Step 6:

STEP 6: Stand with balance on one foot. Find your Triangle and put even pressure on all three corners of it (while maintaining even hips — each hip the same distance from the ground). If you need to, place your hands on a stable surface for support (e.g. table, chair, wall). Returning your feet to the ground like this is the perfect way to cap off the five steps listed above—by standing on your foundation and creating as much stability there as possible.

At every opportunity, practice finding your Triangle and performing these supportive movements. If you're the type who needs an appointment, schedule a time when you can work on your Triangle, and *show up* for your appointment with your feet. Norm and I have found that watching other people — noticing the way they stand, the way their feet are positioned — helps us check in with what *our own* feet are doing at any given moment.

BEING IN NEUTRAL

Among our many goals as educators is to set a new standard for "hip distance." Try this:

After performing Step 6 (above), stand with both feet on the ground. Find your strongest, most balanced position. Your feet are four to six inches apart, pointing straight forward, with weight evenly distributed across your two Triangles. We call this being "on top of your Triangles." From here, we can develop the feeling of what we call "being in neutral."

When standing, our knees and hips should be aimed in the same direction as our feet—straight ahead. When your toes are pointed out (like mine were during my long runs with Norm back in the day), your *knees* turn out, too, which can cause all sorts of problems. Take a moment or two each day to ask yourself: What are my feet and knees doing right now? What do they do when I sit down? When I stand? Are they still four to six inches apart? Or are they a lot wider than that (which can cause your knees to tilt inward)? Even elite athletes forget the importance of correctly positioned feet.

A simple way to remind yourself of this is to remove your shoes and walk or run on a grassy field, barefoot. Whoever created us designed us to move in this way. Doing something active, while barefoot, strengthens the muscles and ligaments in the feet.

Signs of unstable feet include:

» rolling to the outside or inside of the foot

» pointing our toes in a different direction from where our knees are pointed

» flat feet

» bow legs (knees are wider than the feet) or knock knees (knees are narrower than the hips)

For some people, corrective assistance—orthotics, for example—may be required to solidify the foundation. Wearing orthotics does not have to mean that you stop strengthening and stretching the feet. To the contrary, performing proper foot exercises will help you depend on your orthotics less and less. Those who need an orthotic or arch support usually find that it reduces stress on the ankle and knee. (If it doesn't, consult with the medical professional who prescribed them.)

MOVEMENT IS MEDICINE

Our next goal is to take our new foundation and put it into motion. By aligning straight, symmetric feet, with ankles positioned under the hips, we can start to find the stride length that is appropriate for your body.

We have defined our feet as our foundation, but life may force some individuals to redefine this. Years back, we were given the opportunity to help a young high school student who was born with spina bifida and therefore confined to a wheelchair. His father introduced us. Designing a strength training program for him required redefining his foundation, a new place to start his "stack." We focused on his hip girdle and core and began developing a balance between (a) the left and right side of his body, (b) the front and back "halves" of his body (anterior and posterior), and (c) his shoulder girdle and hip girdle.

The work was tedious for him, but it helped him find another valuable tool: his center of gravity. He learned to hinge at the hip instead of rounding forward along his spine. He realized that his hips would always be beneath him, an assurance that gave him increased strength and control throughout his body. This, in turn, allowed him to identify a lifetime of unsound habits that had developed due to overused arm muscles.

We ensured that *all* of his core muscles (not just his abdominals) were involved by changing the angles of our physical training, and by using cables, elastic bands, and dumbbells. He found an inner strength that he never knew was there. He also found his competitive edge, and began engaging in wheelchair sports. He quickly became one of the top athletes in his age group. His progress accomplished what improved strength and control accomplishes for *everyone*: it touched parts of his life he never expected, and it gave him confidence.

There was definitely a learning curve, however. Everything we did was brand new to him and a bit of an experiment for us. It was yet another chapter in life's education. With every new opportunity to help someone learn about their body, Norm and I gain knew knowledge ourselves.

Structural imbalances, postural issues, recurring pain, or inflammation — the list of things that can go wrong in our beautiful and complex musculoskeletal systems is a long one! As with every unique challenge, establishing control of the foundation was a necessary first step. It's a theme we'll return to often in this book, as we deal with each level of the stack.

Before we completely leave the feet, however, we need to learn a bit about the muscles on top of the foot and how they work with the ankle joint. As we learned earlier, the bottom of the foot is comprised of four layers of muscle that help us stabilize our bodies. The muscles of the ankle help us *mobilize*. To do this, our ankle muscles (which actually start around the mid-shin area) work in close partnership with the muscles on top of our foot, which reach all the way to our toes. Exercises like side steps, walking backwards, or step-ups (onto a stair or box) can reveal whether our lower extremities—the structures at the bottom of our stack—are in alignment.

Try these moves in front of a mirror, especially in the early going. Walking backwards really shows us the importance of foot alignment, step size, and hip distance (feet should be about four to six inches apart). When backward walking becomes comfortable, consistent, and balanced, add new wrinkles: walk backward on your toes, or on your heels (flexing your feet up toward your shin). The former strengthens your arch muscles while the latter addresses the muscles on top of the foot and in the lower leg. Suspend a foot in the air and "draw" big circles in the air using your big toe as your pencil. Switch feet. Switch the direction of your circles.

Performing these exercises in combination will put you in touch with the muscles that form your foundation. Further, these exercises will identify the imbalances that prevent your feet from moving identically to one another. Performed daily, these exercises heighten awareness and create new habits.

YOU'RE GROUNDED

It helps sometimes to review our anatomy. Consider the entire machine we just described—the intricate apparatus between the ground and your knee. Start by visualizing the heel bone (calcaneus), which forms the base of your Triangle. On top of that is the talus bone, the protruding knob that is the foundation of the ankle. Spreading downward from the talus is a line of five thin bones that eventually become our toes. Moving *upward* from the talus are two long, sturdy bones—the tibia and fibula—which form our lower leg. The fibula, on the outside of the lower leg, isn't too involved with the knee but is very interactive with the ankle. The tibia, or shinbone, is one of the stoutest bones of the body and relates directly to the knee while transmitting our body weight to the ankle. This entire bony feat of engineering stabilizes the joints in our feet, ankles, and knees, and provides an anchor for the muscles that move them through their full range of motion.

And then there is the Achilles tendon, one of the longest tendons in the body. It inserts at base of the heel and rises to become part of the calf muscle (gastrocnemius) on the back of your lower leg. The Achilles is crucial, in part, because it becomes vulnerable when the foot muscles do not create a level foundation. If your feet roll to the inside (pronate), or if your arches are weak or have dropped to the ground, the Achilles tendon can be tugged out of alignment with every stride you take. Yet another important reason for developing your Triangle. (Whenever I hear about a person, of any age, who is struggling with recurring knee, hamstring, or Achilles injuries, my first instinct is to ask: *How do they use their feet?*)

The point of this brief anatomy lesson is to emphasize the importance of keeping your stack – and the infinite muscles, ligaments, and tendons that surround it—strong and stable. Only then can your stack do its job. These different structures know their individual tasks, but if we ignore or misuse them, weakness sets in and chaos is the result. Without this mindful awareness, without the ability to visualize your bones properly stacked on one another, gravity takes over. Gravity has been here longer than anyone or anything, and gravity is undefeated.

MOVING ON UP

Lifting our focus above the knees, let's get to know the hip rotator muscles at top of the thigh. Try this:

STEP 1: Stand on a level surface, hips over ankles, shoulders over hips.

STEP 2: Gently rest both hands on a stable surface, using the hands only for balance (not support). During the following movements, distribute your weight evenly across your toe joint line.

STEP 3: POSITION A: With feet aiming straight ahead, perform a standing heel raise (see FINDING YOUR TRIANGLE, above). Do eight repetitions, slowly bending at the toe line (balls of the feet).

STEP 4: POSITION B: Keep your heels hip distance apart, but *rotate your toes outward by using the muscles in your hips.* Perform eight standing heel raises in this position, lowering with control.

STEP 5: POSITION C: Aim your feet forward again. Now keep your *toes* hip distance apart while *rotating your heels outward.* Perform eight standing heel raises in this position, lowering with control.

You can use these exercises to gain awareness of the hips' many jobs. These movements also relieve tightness around the ankles and feet, and strengthen the web of rotator muscles that reside at the top of your thigh bone. Remember: the hip rotators are what change the angle of your feet, not your knees. The only time your knees can rotate is when you have "blown them out" (as Norm the veteran stuntman knows all too well).

As we leave the feet and move our focus higher, keep in mind that the easiest and most enjoyable way to build and strengthen the stack in your lower extremities is to walk on the earth as often as possible. This means grass, dirt, or sand. Take your shoes off! The structures in our hips, legs, and feet were designed to interact with natural, ever-changing surfaces, but over the millennia humans have spent more and more of their days on hard, unforgiving, man-made surfaces like concrete, asphalt, and tile.

Sadly, it's not always easy to find a patch of earth, but when you walk on our planet – instead of the substances we have covered her with – the long list of benefits will be worth the effort.

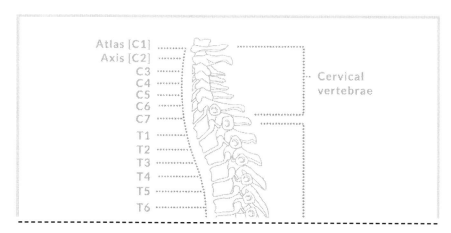

"Anyone can do something when they want to do it. Really successful people do things when they don't want to do it."

– DR. PHIL MCGRAW

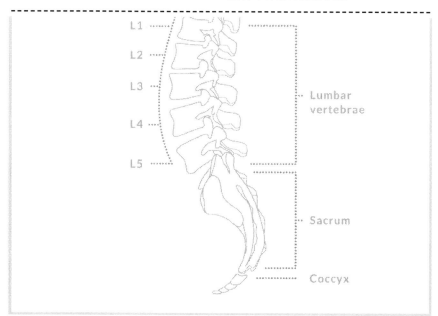

CHAPTER 3
The Wall

ACHIEVING YOUR BEST POSTURE doesn't just refer to the visual aesthetic. Limiting ourselves to what our eyes register ignores the deeper health and wellbeing that can be attained through a well-stacked alignment of our skeleton. The unnecessary stress placed on every system of the body by poor or untrained posture creates issues that can hide within us for years.

Before we move on to the bones and joints that follow the foot and ankle in our upward-moving stack, let's talk about you for a moment. We all have different challenges. All we need is a wall to expose them.

The following postural exercise is both an introduction to Stacking, and a reminder that can be used long after you've begun your journey to better posture.

The Wall Stance:

STEP 1: Stand with your back against a wall, heels against the wall, feet hip distance apart, toes aimed forward. Knees should always be a soft straight never locked.

STEP 2: Place your seat (the most posterior point of your glutes) against the wall.

STEP 3: Place your shoulder blades (scapulae) against the wall.

STEP 4: Relax your neck while allowing your shoulders to drop. Maintain neutral arms with palms facing the body, thumbs facing forward. Do not pull your elbows against the wall.

STEP 5: Gliding your chin backward, keeping your lower jaw parallel with the floor, rest your head against the wall.

During this Wall Stance assessment, we are watching the position of your feet, and looking for a slightly arched lower spine, level hips, and activated abdominal muscles. If this position feels abnormal to you, don't worry, you're not alone. That's what this book is about.

While standing against the wall, keep your focus on a long, relaxed neck—a pedestal for the head to sit on evenly. If these four parts, the feet, hips, shoulder blades, and back of head are touching the wall, congratulations, you're standing straight!

Hold the position for a couple more minutes. Is it hard to maintain? Where do you feel the greatest challenge, the most stress? As you step away from the wall, feel how many muscles were needed to keep your body in posture. Who were the main players? In which muscles do you feel comfort, stability? Which ones are communicating imbalance or weakness?

This assessment, and these questions, cut to the heart of Stacking.

BRICKS IN THE WALL

When all goes well, our side view of the Wall Stance will show ear, shoulder, hip, and ankle alignment. This is our postural goal, for reasons we will discuss throughout this book. That said, each of us is an individual creating his or her own definition of Stacking. Each of us can work positively toward this goal, but we would be wise not to ignore it altogether. Gravity, as we've noted, doesn't take a second off.

From birth, the human body knows how to develop into its strongest, most upright, most balanced individual self. Sometimes, though, we ignore this innate knowledge and allow our environs to dictate our development.

Think for a moment about the way an infant instinctively goes through the stages that end with balanced, controlled walking. We develop from infant to walking toddler because our musculoskeletal system craves activation, craves challenge. Babies naturally seek out tests of their own strength and fitness. Picture a baby working diligently to roll over from his back to his front, strengthening and educating the muscles that help him rotate. His next step is to rock on his hands and knees before embarking on that first, determined crawl. This soon progresses to the curious desire to pull up on anything that will help him get his feet beneath him. Witness his first focused steps away from that support. Walking.

This, of course, is followed by a lifetime of change and challenge and adjustment as the being that was once a baby proceeds through life. When our childhood development ends, the body needs strategic, intentional challenges to keep joints, spine, and feet strong while preserving a balanced Stack.

Our external lives and lifestyles dictate so much to us. Unfortunately, if you are one of those who allows the weight of everyday life to control how you stand (or walk, or sit) you will find the Wall Stance unnatural and challenging to hold for any length of time. And that's okay, for now. Those who find the wall stance easy and natural are in the minority.

Years of ignoring tight muscles or failing to recognize improper foot or spine alignment—these habits make the Wall Stance difficult. When young people are not taught about their bodies' postural needs, growth spurts can end up shaping the way they resist gravity. When your body no longer trusts your ability to do what's best for it, compensations set in and your quality of life becomes less than optimal. Simple movements like walking or getting up from the ground—these are elementary actions that, if ignored, you will one day lose.

Anthropology has proven that our bodies are designed to run, jump, skip, move laterally—the whole athletic gamut. But no matter how old we are, we should also be able to sit or move comfortably while on a flat floor.

Which reminds me of one of my favorite personal stories.

My mother was one of Jack LaLanne's first followers. I'll always remember coming home from school to find Mom with her personal trainer "Jack" on TV. My mother's posture was balanced long before she knew how important it was. She stayed physically active and flexible throughout her life. Even in her 70s, I'd find her sitting cross-legged on her bathroom counter, putting on make-up in front of the mirror. She had strength, flexibility, and graceful control of her spine muscles. She kept her joints healthy. Good posture was something she aspired to, and taught, for her whole life. Not because of the science we now have, but because of the inner instinct she possessed that told her this was important.

A BRIEF ANATOMY LESSON

The skeletal system is basically divided into two groups: the (1) "axial skeleton," the skull, vertebrae, sternum, and ribs (a sturdy, core group surrounded by muscles, ligaments and tendons that hold these bones in position), and the (2) "appendicular skeleton," which includes the bones of the arms, hands, legs, and feet, plus the shoulder and pelvic girdles.

It's amazing how each bone, each joint, knows its role. At a certain point in our lives, however, we are faced with a new task—that of making sure these bones stay positioned in their pockets. We do this in order to (1) allow full range of motion and (2) ward off injury and imbalance. The focus, as always, is function. The shape of the body is a by-product of quality function.

When your bones are in their pockets, they're in their strongest position. This minimizes friction and wear-and-tear in the tissues that surround the joints. This also lets the ligaments, tendons and muscles be at their natural lengths. "Pocketed" bones contribute to a strong spine, and allow the proper space for our organs to do their work. They also create overall symmetry—the right side mirroring the left—and greater bone density. Proper posture perfects the natural leverages that are handed to us at birth.

Many of us think that physical pain and weakness are signs of normal aging. Not true. It's our lack of awareness, our inability to identify our own sub-par body positioning, that brings pain and movement limitations to our Stack. Over-compensations usually follow, resulting in deeper challenges.

In some cases, an individual can appear to be doing all the right things when pain and limited movement strike. Some of us deal with postural issues that began before birth—for example: me and my scoliosis—yet we don't realize there's an issue until pain shows up to tell us. Once we're informed of this unfortunate fact, the next step should be to seek out a diagnosis by a professional, which may include an x-ray or MRI. Only with an informed diagnosis can you start rebuilding your Stack.

A lot can be learned on the floor of a gym or fitness center, just by watching and listening to the people who frequent such places. Some of these folks try to duplicate a group of exercises they saw online, or copy whatever they see other people in the gym doing. Without a complete assessment to determine one's imbalances, structural issues, and individual goals, attempting random exercises is, more often than not, followed by injury. The starting point afforded by our Stacking assessments (Finding Your Triangle, for example, or The Wall Stance) can be revisited later to help determine whether you're making progress or creating more chaos.

I was unaware of having scoliosis in my upper thoracic spine until different types of discomfort, pain, and tightness surfaced. This warning began with tightness in my neck that traveled down to my upper back. As we age, our body can start losing the cushioning between vertebrae and other joints, as mine did. My pain ultimately settled in my left shoulder. When this pain began interfering with my life, I went to see two orthopedists. After multiple x-rays I was told that there was an imbalance in strength. Physical therapy was prescribed. I knew my body well enough to know this was not the cause of my pain, but I gave their suggestion a try. PT didn't help.

Fortunately, I was referred to a third orthopedic surgeon who expanded on the previous exams and tried new x-ray positions. My issue was exposed: the abnormal curvature at the top of my spine had reduced the space between two important bones near my shoulder. Because the inflammation and pain were increasing, I elected surgery.

Surgery reduced the length of the bones and smoothed a couple of pesky bone spurs. My normal range of motion returned. I returned to my active life with a new awareness. The ensuing physical therapy supported this awareness and furthered my personal education. Surgery and therapy did not remove my scoliosis, but it did allow me to discover new ways to find balance and strength, without pain. I had always strived to keep my body strong; now I had a new way of assessing strength. Our belief is: Do not live in pain when there is most likely a solution!

Again: pain doesn't need to be an accepted step in the aging process. If left undiagnosed and unaddressed, pain will reduce movement and bring about a compensation. The ensuing wear and tear and inflammation will cause even more chaos. Not everything that causes pain requires surgery. An accurate diagnosis, however, will provide you with the best place to start.

BALANCING ACT

My new knowledge about my spine and neck began the lengthier process of finding new tools to balance and strengthen all my joints, including those in my spine and feet. Traditional resistance training was not helping my situation, but continuing to irritate and inflame it. My spine could not allow an exercise involving compression. This is usually between the shoulder girdle and hips or the hips and soles of feet. The reason is simple...the left and right sides of my spine did not match. My crooked hip girdle affected the way my feet interacted with the ground. I needed to train my limbs and opposing sides separately.

An old exercise known as the "Farmers Walk," which involves holding a weight (usually a kettle or dumb bell) in one hand while walking with neutral and level posture, provided a huge benefit and a versatile training tool that safely targeted my spine. By taking this concept of "unbalanced loads" and adding it to our lunges, squats, and core workouts, we realized we were onto something. This unbalanced approach seemed especially helpful to those who were new to strength training or who had chronic imbalances. To the seasoned athlete, it brought balance and awareness of space.

Combined with postural Stacking, this approach has brought pain relief to many of our friends and clients over the years. It provided balance within the body's three planes of movement: front/back, top/bottom, left/right.

Through the years, we've had several clients with scoliosis (in various parts of the spine). One client had an abnormal curve in her sternum. After suffering from extreme shoulder pain, she underwent surgery to repair a small muscle tear and smooth some bone spurs. We later learned that her doctor did not take her sternum and neck into consideration. So now, years later, the shoulder continues to have imbalances and is always trying to adjust. She is able to live an active lifestyle, but the shoulder will probably always require neck and rotator cuff therapy.

Each case of scoliosis is marked by pain in the areas above and/or below the breakdown in our vertebral Stack. Pain is not always felt in the area of the breakdown. Rather, it's a symptom, a warning that something is amiss.

As nice as it is to have balanced strength, we must also strive for balanced flexibility. Many adults include yoga or Pilates in their programs, which we feel are extremely beneficial when taught with individual needs in mind. Some positions are not for everyone. Body awareness, foot control, and a strong core and posture must come first. These three basics give us the ability to know when we're going somewhere that could harm a joint or compromise our posture. Each person's Stack is as unique as his or her fingerprint, so remember: resist the urge to compare yourself to the shapes, routines, and abilities of others.

The Wall Stance is most difficult for those with tight, unbalanced muscles. The most common failings with the Wall Stance are (1) an inability to rest the head against the wall, (2) no arch in the lower spine, and (3) too much arch in the lower spine. Those who struggle to keep their heels against the wall usually have a lower rib cage that protrudes forward and palms that rotate backward (facing behind you). Remember: learning to move with a balanced Stack, in all directions, is our goal. As we continue to discuss the functions and structural relationships within the Stack, the clarity with which you'll see the need to strengthen and lengthen the involved muscles will sharpen. Better posture is great, but we are seeking improved function within our new posture. A perfect Stack is worthless if it crumbles when in motion.

This is why we advise against using exercise machines. It is common to have opposing joints, hinges, or bone lengths that aren't symmetrical (i.e. don't match). When this is the case, the last thing your body wants is to be confined by a device. Using dumbbells, bands, cables, medicine balls, and your own body weight are better choices as you develop your new control and awareness. We cannot stress it enough: not every exercise is appropriate for everyone—not even squats, as universal as that old standby may seem.

STACKING IN ACTION

When choosing exercises, you first want to identify the weak or unbalanced areas, then, using strong, balanced feet as your foundation, constantly check in with your Triangle as you work. Squats, power cleans, deadlifts, and other multi-joint exercises can be useful, but only after your foundation—the building blocks of body aware-ness—has been constructed first.

Here's an example of someone who came to us needing help with multiple issues, all at the same time. (This is the case with most persons seeking postural help.) An avid golfer was referred to us, post-rehab, when efforts to address his lower back pain showed no results. The comments we received from his physical therapist consisted of: "needs to continue to strengthen core." X-rays and an MRI showed no struc-tural issues, which demonstrated to us, once again, that just because your imaging looks good doesn't mean your skeletal alignment is on point. We knew just from observing him that his main issue was a Stacking issue.

At our first consultation, the most prominent breakdowns were easily visible. Even before he did the Wall Stance, his natural walking gait showed that he walked on the outside edges of his feet, with toes turned in. His upper leg tracked down wider than his hip line and his lower leg tracked up outside his ankle/heel – which is a fancy way of saying: He had bow legs.

Even with this limitation, he was still capable of building a solid Stack. But he also had a torso that leaned forward at the waist, com-pounding an already tight hinge line at the hips. His elbows were habitually pulled back, causing a tight upper back and a head that sat ahead of his shoulders, extending his neck.

When he stood against the wall, we saw (see if any of this applies to you): his lower back arch extended all the way to his shoulder blades, his head could not touch the wall, his shoulders could not sit natu-rally with palms turned toward his body. We began with a balanced approach focused on simple things: the stretching and strengthening of the bottoms of his feet and ankles; movements to develop matching hips, knees, ankles, and feet (Triangles). We built the bottom floors first. As his range of motion increased, he learned to use his hips instead of his waist. Lateral movements and lunges strengthened and stretched long-ignored gluteal muscles.

Every physically compromised person requires his or her own specialized training program, so we're not prescribing specific exercises here. The general idea, though—with this client and with most others—is a circuit-type training program that strengthens the core and increases and makes symmetrical the ranges of motion in the shoulder girdle and neck muscles. As you probably guessed, the main work is to develop a relationship between the bottom of the foot, the knee, and the hip. We did not change the shape of his bow legs—we're not orthopedic surgeons—but we did develop the muscle support, one limb at a time, that is required to carry uneven loads and to delegate work to the various muscles surrounding each joint.

The simple information gained from the Wall Stance was priceless to this process. None of this is rocket science. Movement, rather, is an art. Even simple moves like sitting down and standing up correctly can be life changing. Our ailing golfer, by the way, is no longer in pain, and in fact has taken up competitive stand-up paddle boarding. He is over 70 years old. His decision to heal himself would never have paid off without his tenacity, competitive spirit, and patience. With those three traits, a person can accomplish just about anything.

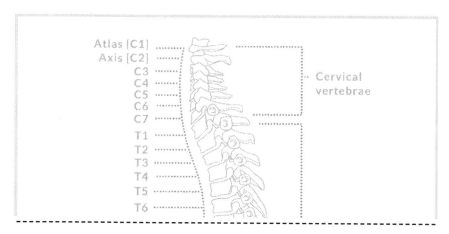

"Don't let what you cannot do interfer with what you can do."

- JOHN WOODEN

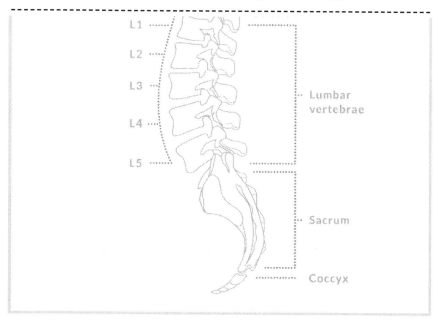

CHAPTER 4
Knees and Hips

Nancy vs. Knee Replacement:

"I tore my cartilage in both knees when I was in high school. After that I remember that if I went down stairs too quickly one of my knees would go out and swell. Then I would favor it for about 6 weeks until it healed. When I was in my early 50s I noticed both knees were becoming thicker. I had an MRI and was told I had arthritis in both knees and I would need replacements eventually. My left knee also had a loose body in it, which would act up and feel painful. I heard about Debbie from my son, who went to the gym she worked from. Debbie immediately helped me to strengthen the muscles around my knees and worked on my feet and distributing my weight correctly on my feet, which helped my knees. She gave me specific exercises and showed me the correct way to place my knees and feet when I walked. I had gotten to the point that I could not get off the ground from sitting position without help. Debbie showed me the correct way, along with strengthening technique, that allowed me to do this without pain. That was liberating for me! This included the posturing and core control. I feel like I have new knees and since doing this work I have not had one instance of my knee "going out." I am 65 years old and this is the best my knees have been since I was 16! I am so grateful she was able to help me."

The tibia, also known as the shin bone, is the stoutest bone in the body. It transfers body weight from the knee to the ankle and provides a stage where the patella (kneecap) and femur (thigh bone) connect with it and work as a three-bone team. With this huge responsibility, and because the knee is the stabilizing point, having balance, integrity, and alignment within the knee-tibia and tibia-ankle relationships is a must.

To visualize this part of your Stack, think of your feet as two commanders who give orders to the ankles and knees above them. Whatever direction the foot turns, the knee follows. This relationship, of course, is transferred up the femur (thigh) and into the hip joint.

The hip has six deep rotator muscles lying beneath the gluteal muscles. The work of these hidden (but incredibly strong) muscles affects our feet more than most of us realize. Which is why, when there's an imbalance in the hip, it shows up in the Triangle, too. Most untrained eyes can see such imbalances just by standing in front of a mirror.

When we think of the four quadriceps muscles and three hamstring muscles in the thigh, we usually think of them in terms of sports or sports injuries. But athletics is merely a glittery stage for these workhorses. Their more important job gets done with no fanfare, when they are helping provide stability, balance—and protective padding, in some instances—to the all-important knee and hip joints.

REPLACING JOINT REPLACEMENT

To allow our bodies to age into a lifestyle that is both active and independent (there's no law that says you have to use a walker at age 80), we have to maintain the integrity of these crucial hip and knee joints by remaining active. In later years, this activity is only possible when a strong balanced Stack is in place to support it, with each bone resting in its pocket.

Among our greatest joys has been the positive feedback we've gotten from friends and clients who at one point were facing a knee or hip replacement. (Many of these referrals came about because of Norm's "hands-on research"—a.k.a. injuries—as a Hollywood stunt man.) The most common challenges we see are damaged ligaments or cartilage in the knee, which often results in a dreaded "bone-on-bone" situation. Some of these folks were told that they would never run or jump again and that surgery is just "buying time until knee replacement." With all due respect to the doctors who blindly offer such prognoses, Norman is still running, sprinting, jumping, and lunging—and he does so on a knee that is bone on bone. The difference is that he has put in the work necessary to stabilize that joint by strengthening the muscles surrounding it. (Check out his YouTube video: Senior Parkour.)

We love it when our colleagues in the orthopedic world tell us, "Whatever you're doing, don't stop." But all we've done is find ways to stabilize our knees and hips. Sure, most of this work occurs in the gym, but it also includes surfing, rollerblading, and walking in the sand together, shooting the breeze and focusing on our Triangles. We are honored to have become the "go-to persons" in our small beach community for those hoping to either avoid a joint replacement or to learn to live with one. To thrive with one.

Cardio alone does not get it done when the goal is to build the knee and hip sections of your Stack. Programs that consist solely of monotonous cardio often do more harm than good. Cross training (not to be confused with CrossFit) provides a better choice than cardio due to the multiple angles and movements presented. The goal is to involve as many muscles as possible, with as many different (yet safe) movements that require the feet, ankles, knees, and hips, to work both together and independently of one another. The best training recipes call for just the right dose of unpredictability.

Some of the less "sexy" work includes holding a Wall Stance while focusing on the details described in Chapter 3. The Wall Stance will tell you if your hip hinge has fallen behind your ankle bone. It will alert you when your knees are locked or when your feet are wider than your hips. The health and function of the knee is dependent on the development of an even, balanced gait—and that starts with the feet. Similarly, the health of the spine depends in large part on shoulder and hip alignment. This, too, gets exposed by the Wall Stance.

Simply feeling your Triangle on the bottom of your foot is the first step toward strengthening the muscles in your lower leg. The tall muscles at the front of your shin are there to pull your foot (specifically the Triangle line along the balls of your feet) up toward your chin. This action allows the ankle to rock. Walking provides lots of exercise to these anterior shin muscles, but remember what we said earlier about the need for new challenges. When this need is ignored, especially in middle age, we risk waking up one day to discover that we are merely shuffling instead of walking.

Here's an example of the way the dozens of muscles in your foot work together. Start in a seated position (preferably on the floor, but a chair or ottoman are fine if the floor isn't comfortable). Keep the foot flat on the floor, aimed straight ahead so that the toes stay aligned with the kneecap.

STEP 1: extend the foot at the ankle, pointing your toes like a ballerina. Focus on squeezing your arch. With the ankle locked in this extended position, pull the toes back as far as possible, then back to pointing.

STEP 2: bring the top of the foot back toward the shin bone by bending at the ankle.

THE LEG: AN AMAZING MACHINE

The muscles in the back of the lower leg help us push the ground away when we're in motion. There are about four layers of muscles connecting the ankle to the knee, but the two that do most of the work are the gastrocnemius (commonly referred to as the calf muscle) and the soleus (which lies somewhat hidden beneath its more famous partner). The most obvious way to challenge these muscles is with heel raises. These are done by standing and lifting your body onto the balls of your feet (we call it the toe line) by moving only your ankle joint. Advanced exercisers can do these one leg at a time.

While we usually identify these two muscle layers as relating to the foot and ankle, they also play a role in (a) preventing an unsafely locked knee and (b) stabilizing the knee joint in general.

The inside of the knee consists of ligaments, tendons, and cartilage that – working in many different directions – stabilize and cushion the joint, allowing all of the different ranges of motion we demand from it. But these soft tissues have their limits. The larger ligaments surround the inner knee and work with the stabilizers and cushions. If the involved muscles aren't in control and doing their job, it doesn't take much to damage a ligament. As many of us know, everyday, unathletic, normal life can bring harm to this area.

What usually happens is that the foot plants, pointing forward, while the knee twists inward. Climbing or descending stairs while distracted is a common way to injure the knee's soft tissues. General muscular weakness in the area can allow the knees to lock or even hyperextend (bend backward). Simply rising from a chair without properly engaging the knee can have unwelcome consequences.

Remember, these are very small connective tissues with very big responsibilities. After a certain amount of misuse—pop—they are forced to give in. This most often results in an ACL or meniscus injury. We've had two individuals sent to us following surgery to repair a torn meniscus. Neither of them understood what they had done because they never exercised and thus were out of touch with their body's structures. That's another common way to get hurt: lack of exercise.

Injury prevention in the knee and hip areas includes knowing and maintaining the relationship between the foot's Triangle and the knee, and keeping that relationship intact through the upper leg, into the hip. Know this: the body wants to communicate and react as one unit. To allow this, we have to keep our mind/body connections alive by giving them the appropriate attention, and yes, the appropriate work.

The stack is moved by muscle groups, not individual muscles. The upper leg muscles that end at the knee (quads, hamstrings) also come together within the hip girdle. But they aren't there alone. Along with the six deep rotators we mentioned earlier, there are three thick gluteal muscles that run in different directions. As any orthopedist will tell you, these gluteals have a direct effect on the health of the lower spine.

Posturally speaking, the most important interaction among all of these muscles is their ability (or inability) to stabilize the hinge where the leg and hip connect. The human hip joint is a fascinating apparatus that (a) moves in multiple directions, (b) mobilizes the leg (a heavy, complex appendage) and (c) provides a foundation for the spine and torso. The hip movements most people think about are walking, running, or jumping. But performing those movements isn't enough if you want to keep your hips strong and ward off low back pain.

As with the feet and ankles, you don't have to "go heavy" when training the hips; rather, the goal should be to move the joint in all directions. Walking backward, side-stepping, doing a carioca step (or "grapevine" as we called it in dance and aerobics), where you repeatedly cross your legs while moving sideways—these are easy and effective ways to keep the hips mobile.

Here are two more: (1) stand, lift one leg, and make big circles in the air with one foot, then the other; (2) in a kneeling or all-fours position, circle one bent knee at a time. Remember, if there's a muscle there's a reason.

The most natural response when moving or exercising is to consider only those muscles that we can see or feel working; for example the large upper leg muscles, or the calves. But as with the muscles on the bottom of the foot, the hip has important layers of muscle working beneath the surface.

GET MOVING

Leading a sedentary life will sooner or later create imbalances. And today's humans are more sedentary than ever.

The human body is meant to move. Think about all the little joints and hinges we need to do even the simplest movements: walking, sitting, carrying a bag, climbing stairs, bending to pick something up. The long-term integrity of these connections depends on you. To keep these simple movements in your life as you age, you have to remain active. Move it or lose it. Some of these movements are so easy that they eliminate laziness as an excuse. Working with your bodyweight and a few bands usually provides enough resistance in the beginning, but the safe addition of moderate weights, imbalanced weights, or an elevated surface, will help you add integrity and stability to your body.

Over the years I have heard hundreds of people ask how they can find relief from lower back pain. In severe cases, I always confirm my assessment with what's visible on x-rays or MRIs. In a majority of cases, the culprit is an imbalance in the gluteal muscles. The shape and size of these muscles are as unique as their angles of action and the locations of their connections to surrounding bones. As with the feet, the importance of this area is vastly underrated. A lack of balanced Stacking in the hip girdle creates chaos and dysfunction at the hinge, which hinders mobility and results in poor posture.

Too many of us bend forward using the middle of our spine, or our waist, instead of our hip hinge. Over time, this becomes a "new normal." We've met so many people who considered themselves fit (and across most of their body, they were), only to have the Wall Stance expose the surprising truth: that their glutes and hip rotators had atrophied.

THE HIPS: OUR PRIME MOVERS

The average person either doesn't use or doesn't know how to use over half of their hip muscles. This condition causes some of the larger muscles near the hip (including the hamstrings and erector spinae [lower back] muscles) to become overloaded. Maintaining solid posture while performing the simple hip movements described in this chapter will help break these harmful patterns and "re-teach" the hip how to move. Stay aware of your recently discovered Triangle and the tibia-knee connection above it; that's where hip health starts!

A note about flexibility: the hip hinge functions poorly when the muscles around it are tight. Inflexible hips are another common cause of lower back pain, which is why, when we begin working with an individual who has Stacking issues, the hip hinge is among the first areas we assess.

Bad habits in the hips can be hard to break. A new client came to us with pain and chronic inflammation in the right side of her low back. We addressed the imbalance with a plan that started with her Triangles, then moved inch by inch into her hips, then her core. In the beginning, she was so stiff and in so much pain that she couldn't exercise for very long at all. We used this downtime to analyze her daily habits. We asked her to demonstrate how she got in and out of her car. That wasn't the issue, we learned. We looked at the way her legs were positioned when driving; again, not the cause. Same with her sleeping position; it was fine. By this point we were getting a little frustrated. What were we missing? What was causing these issues?

Finally, we analyzed the way she sat at her desk at work. Bingo. This was a petite woman, 5 feet tall, and her desk was too high for her chair. To compensate, she'd been tucking her right leg beneath her hip, to lift herself slightly higher when seated.

Her hip rotators and glutes had been compressed and overstretched for ... who knows how long. (She had held the same job for years.) No wonder she had back pain. We explained to her what we found and advised her to sit on a firm pillow at work and put her feet on a stool. Soon afterward, her back pain stopped.

But that was only half the battle. Now she had to bring her body back to balance. We helped her reshape the dominant muscle groups and encouraged her to find a new awareness of what "level" felt like at the hips! Which brings us back to the Triangle. Even when you're seated with your feet on the ground, feeling your Triangle can give the knees guidance. That alignment rises into the hips and teaches the hip hinge to remain neutral.

Humans love to use advanced age as an excuse to limit our movements. As we get older, we tend to move around less, which can cause our physical challenges (weakness, poor balance) to spread into other areas of our lives. When we stop moving, we deny our bodies a chance to strengthen these shortcomings.

Norm and I can't tell you how often we hear our friends say things like, "I didn't even see it coming ... It all happened so fast ... One day, I was ... old!" One of our first questions for those near or past middle age is: Can you rise from the floor?

It's a dark day when you find yourself afraid to sit or lie on the ground, when you no longer trust your ability to rise from there. Seeing a 50-year-old (or 70-year-old, for that matter) who is hesitant to step up onto a curb for fear of tripping and falling is just as heartbreaking. We don't have to fear getting older. We can age and do all the things we once did if we maintain a base level of strength and balance (and maintain a manageable body weight).

Are you prepared for an unforeseen stumble? Can you react in time to prevent a fall, or limit the impact from a fall? Are you able to rise from the ground afterward? We're raising these questions now because we have only discussed the lower half of the body. It's time to continue building your Stack at the spine.

And if you think the abilities to descend to the ground and rise from it aren't important, ask yourself: Where will your youngest grandchildren play?

You got it, on the floor.

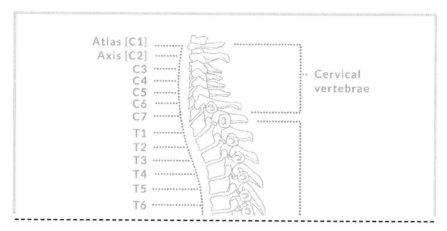

"If it's important, you'll find a way. If not, you'll find an excuse."

- JIM ROH

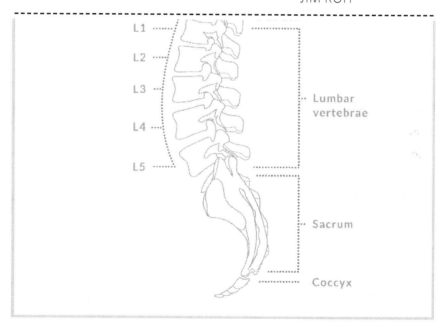

CHAPTER 5
Spine

CONGRATULATIONS, we're at the halfway mark—of both this book, and your body's vertical structure. We've arrived at the spine.

You have learned so far that to build a human skeleton, the Triangle on the bottom of your foot is your stabilizing foundation. Our ankle and knee needs direction on how to move—or how to stay put—and our Triangles give us just that. All of this allows the hip girdle to have its normal function. Do you recognize the pattern?

Stabilizing.

Mobilizing.

Stabilizing.

Mobilizing.

Let's keep building our Stack.

The spine is made up of a chain of 24 small bones, each with a unique shape and a hole in its center through which the spinal cord carries its crucial, lightning-fast terabytes of information. The spine is widely considered the most important part of our bodies, due to its irreplaceable roles in both the nervous and skeletal systems. It provides the structure and support upon which our limbs move. It can also move on its own—rotating, twisting, flexing, extending—in infinite ways. It protects our most vital bundles of nerves. The spine is an intelligent, flowing fortress, which can define a person's strength and integrity. Each of the joints along the spine is one of a kind, an engineering marvel unto itself.

Each of these joints (the 24 vertebrae in the cervical, thoracic, and lumbar region; plus the fused sacral and coccygeal vertebrae at the base of the spine) has a limited range of motion and relies on strong muscles and connective tissue to maintain optimum posture. When the smallest of these links becomes weak and falters, the entire column is compromised, followed by the body itself.

Through the years, many of our friends and clients have had challenges that required adjustments in their Stack. Life's potholes and collisions had left many of them with rods, pins, artificial joints, and all the damage the spine is susceptible to. Unless these dented bodies address the feet and ankles, however, everything between the knees and shoulders remains vulnerable. Tightness always wins in the absence of work to release that tightness and move in our full ranges of motion. Tight muscles won't loosen up on their own; they will only get tighter. The spine is no exception. In fact, based on the all-too-common complaint of "lower back pain," the spine offers the greatest example of this rule. Traditional physical therapy can help relieve tightness and immobility in the spine, but unless this work is integrated with the rest of the body, imbalances will almost certainly strike again.

LIFESTYLES OF THE STACKED AND (NOT NECESSARILY) FAMOUS

The daily habits of our 21st-Century lifestyles can adversely shape our spines unless we counter them with brief periods of alignment-focused exercise. This does not require one hour per day, or even 30 minutes, and the benefits far outweigh the time it takes to keep your spine healthy and strong.

The consequences of poor posture can start at a very young age. Most of us are not taught of the spine's importance until problems arise. The most common issue, in our experience, arises when we use different sections of the spine as a hinge or bending point without developing the necessary muscular support. Lifting items with a "rounded back" is perhaps the most obvious example. The center of your spine is not meant to bear a heavy load by itself, hence the age-old advice: Lift with your legs. When you feel that first spasm, or when you sense that you're asking too much of this durable column of bone, soft tissue, and nerves, that's when it's time to take a step back, refocus, and find yourself a wall.

There are layers of muscles, long and short, that support and control the infinite ranges of motion in your spine. There are deeper layers of muscle that aren't visible when looking at an unclothed human back. They work in secret, like the steel girders of a skyscraper, which never see the light of day after they're covered in cement. One such group of muscles is the erector spinae in the lower back, a web of thick muscle that connects the pelvis, vertebrae, and ribs and extends all the way to the neck and head. These deep muscles are a common source of pain because of how often we use them—and misuse them. If we remain mobile, flexible and properly "Stacked," however, the undue stress on the erector spinae can be all but eliminated.

Farther from the ground lie the larger muscles of the upper back, which control the spine's relationship with the shoulder girdle. The trapezius, rhomboids, and latissimus, along with a few other muscles around the shoulder blades and neck, control our arm movements. Again, it's not important to memorize the names of all these muscles; there won't be a quiz later. Acknowledging them, however, helps us understand the layers and complexities involved in maintaining a healthy spine. This understanding allows for proper "Stacking." Strengthening the large, superficial muscles without paying attention to the deeper ones, will bring instability. Every good architect knows that making renovations on a 100-year-old home requires that the aging building's skeleton be taken into account at every turn.

SPINES NEED FLEXIBILITY TOO!

Above, we touched upon the dangers of using the mid-spine as a hinge, a lever. A stronger, safer option is to use the deep lower back muscles in conjunction with the hamstrings. This is the way we are designed to move. Here are a couple of stretches that will not only be relaxing but, as we learned with the wall stance, they'll reveal imbalances.

For the first one, sit on the floor next to a wall, with your legs straight in front of you and your spine and tailbone pressed against the wall. Keeping your legs straight, widen your feet to greater than hip distance apart; your toes are still pointing straight up at the ceiling or sky. From this position, the goal is to be able to lean forward with a neutral spine—straight yet relaxed—with the hip crease as your main hinge. The tailbone remains stationary and "glued to the floor." The head and chest are neutral or slightly lifted as you lean forward. Avoid the temptation to bend forward somewhere along your spine; aka, "hump back."

Lean forward from your hinge.

There will be different starting points for each of you. For some, just keeping the legs straight and toes pointed up will be a good start. We cannot reiterate how fine this is. No one is competing here. We are Stacking. It took thirty years to build the Washington Monument. Be patient with yourself.

The second stretch, below, helps with tightness in all the leg muscles, as well as those in the low back.

Lie on your side, with your feet near a flat wall. While staying on your side, move your glutes toward the wall until they touch. Swing both legs up, to 12 o'clock, so that the hamstrings, calves and heels are touching the wall and the soles of your feet are aimed at the sky. You should look like the letter L with your torso on the ground and legs up on the wall. (Some are not able to keep their glutes on the wall at first due to muscle tightness, but with time and consistent practicing of this stretch, this tightness will decrease, allowing your rear to get closer to the wall and create that true L.)

Now: with your spine on the floor, feeling lengthened and relaxed, spread your arms out wide, like an eagle, palms facing the ceiling. Allow your legs to widen an inch or two every thirty seconds or so. Keep the ankles and feet relaxed. Hold for a minimum of one minute. Three to five minutes would be optimum.

Both of these stretches will not only loosen the tightness throughout your spine, it will put you in connection with your hip hinge and lower back.

MINDFUL EXERCISE

Let's switch gears for a moment. Through the years, one of the most common health behaviors we see is attempting to lose weight via extreme dieting and extreme quantities of cardio. First, these well-meaning souls restrict their caloric intake, which is a bad way to start due to the inadequate hydration and nutrient intake that comes as a result. Next, they pile tons of cardio on themselves. Let's hope they have at least a general understanding of posture and balance at this point, or else they're in trouble. With luck, they will know the importance of starting with the feet. Without these two tenets, cardio work will bring more pain than results.

Think of it this way: a runner takes approximately 2,000 strides when running a mile. If we choose this kind of highly repetitive activity for our cardio, the position of the foot each time it makes contact with the ground determines the control of every joint or hinge above it. When we add your body weight to the equation, things can get rough, especially if the feet and ankles aren't stacked properly. If you drive your car on a flat tire for long distances, will your suspension and alignment be adversely affected? Absolutely. Where our bodies are concerned, the most common results of distance running (or walking) on mis-stacked feet are knee pain and low back pain.

Remember your Triangle. Your spine will reap the benefits.

Now put your newfound awareness of this feet-spine connection into practice. If you retain nothing else from this book, hold onto these two nuggets:

Start with the feet.

Everything is connected.

When walking or running, the feet are the only body parts that touch the ground. (As opposed to other exercise choices like push-ups, yoga, or swimming [where nothing touches the ground!]). The feet are your points of control. This control is based not only on how each foot lands, but where the toes are pointing. A properly planted foot gives the knees, hips, and core—and the hundreds of tendons, ligaments, and muscle fascia—the power to move safely and efficiently. Consider your "arm swing" as well. When walking, keep your shoulders directly above your hips and move your arms like two smooth-arcing pendulums, each flowing in time with the opposite leg.

INFLAMMATION NATION

Earlier, we mentioned a client who had developed lower back pain but didn't realize it was due to an overcompensation that followed an ankle injury. This is an example of how all the limbs, hinges and joints affect the health of the ones above and below. After injuring his ankle, this client developed a new walk that protected the ankle by keeping it as immobile as possible. Imagine the effect of wearing a walking boot for the rest of your life. Do you think your hips and spine would suffer? Of course they would.

This client, not realizing the importance of physical therapy, allowed inflammation to move in for an extended stay. The lack of movement in the ankle meant less movement at the bottom of the foot. His knee became less mobile, as well, which meant that the hip was solely responsible for lifting the leg and moving it forward, into the next step. Low back pain resulted because the spine was no longer resting on a level hip girdle. Inflammation took over from there, creating a loss of arch in the lumbar (low back) region and increased tightness in the thoracic (mid back) region. The final score:

Weakness and Imbalance: 1

Client: 0

During our meetings with this client, a solution began to take shape. We returned to the Triangle, strengthening the bottom of the foot and stretching the muscles that had become hazardously tight. We did seated, non-weight bearing rotational work with his ankle—asking him to move his toes from 10 o'clock to 2 o'clock, and back again, using only the ankle joint. As this foundational work progressed, we moved to the hip, performing simple tasks like balancing on one foot. This balance work brought the core muscles into play, the result of which was more support for the lower spine. To allow for new adjustments and freedoms, we integrated a stretching routine that employed all of the different ranges of motion. Slowly, his ankle joint got involved again, reintroducing itself to the hinges above and below it. By this time, the client's low back pain had subsided dramatically.

Which brings us to the topic of inflammation.

Inflammation is defined by the Merriam-Webster dictionary as "a local response to cellular injury that is marked by capillary dilatation ... redness, heat, and pain." Inflammation causes stress on our bodies on many levels. Where our Stacking efforts are concerned, inflammation can prevent bones from lining up and "sitting" in the pockets where they're designed to sit.

One of the most important steps toward recovering from an injury or surgery is physical therapy. In fact, we believe that completing a well-designed PT program is the first step to full recovery. Failure to complete PT (saying, "I feel better, I don't need to do the rest of this stuff") or worse, not doing any PT at all, usually brings negative results, including increased inflammation. In the realm of therapy and healing, we believe that seeing things through until the end is a must. The only exception is a program that is causing undue pain or is worsening the condition. Otherwise, do the work!

It's also important to remember, Stackers, that if you're doing rehab exercises for one limb, repeat them on the opposite side to maintain balance during the healing process. No human has ever been 100 percent symmetrical, but our goal is to strive for harmony and physical equilibrium by treating one side the same as the other during therapy.

THE SACRED SACRUM

Your spinal column is round and snakelike, but each segment has a different shape. Some vertebrae are thicker in the anterior (front) section; others are thicker in the posterior. The combination of these shapes allows for better weight-bearing and function, and gives the spine its distinctive, curved S shape. At the bottom of this S is the sacrum, a triangular bone comprised of five fused vertebrae that sits between the two hipbones. The sacrum transfers the weight of the upper body to the hips.

It is difficult to feel this part of the body, and to hold the subtle arch of the lumbar (low back) region, without visualizing it. Here is a position that may help you develop this connection:

Sit on an inflated stability ball with your feet flat on the floor and your knees hip-distance apart. (You can use a chair or bench if a ball isn't available.) In this position, visualize a perfectly shaped spine with your tailbone behind you, not curled under you. Now try and feel what yoga teachers call your "sit bones;" these are the two bones deep within your gluteus muscles that bear your weight when you're sitting with proper posture. Balance your weight evenly on these "sit bones" while gently lifting the rib cage, creating a natural arch in your low back. Don't force it. Don't over-arch your spine. Your shoulders should hover directly above your hips. This position is complete when your chin is parallel with the floor, your eyes are looking forward, the Triangle beneath each foot is in firm, relaxed contact with the ground, and you are breathing comfortably.

Stability in the all-important low back/hip area involves a strong working relationship between the muscles of the hip girdle and those of the core. All sides of the core, too: left, right, front, and back. The basic tasks we perform on a day-to-day basis—sitting, rising, walking, climbing stairs—depend on this relationship. This dead horse we keep beating is pretty black and blue by now, but guess what: It all starts with the feet. Then the knees. Then hips. These are the foundations of your Stack. These are the lower floors of your skyscraper. Build them with precision and durability in mind.

Upon these lower floors rests the torso, buttressed by all of those multi-dimensional vertebrae, and all of their individual shapes and roles. The five quadrilateral lumbar vertebrae, the lowest and most massive bones of the spinal column, carry a disproportionate share of your body weight, balancing the torso on the sacrum and working with the hips to allow pain-free standing, walking, and running.

Because of the spine's unique mobility and shape—not to mention the vital nerves encased within the vertebrae—strength in the muscles around the spine is necessary to avoid injury. The only thing that keeps the vertebrae in their proper pockets is muscle. Core exercises can be used in many ways—balance work, unbalanced loads, rotational work—that have little to do with the abdominals, the washboard-shaped sheath of muscle behind your navel that are often given undue priority in the gym.

MID-BACK AND UPPER BACK

This brings us to the twelve thoracic vertebrae. This section developed its shape while you were still in the womb. It serves as the anchor for our twenty-four ribs, which protect the heart and lungs and come together on the other side at the sternum (breastbone). Weaving in and out of these twelve vertebrae are supportive muscles that are relatively small and run in different angles. They also help control the position of the shoulder blades and therefore determine the health and strength of the shoulders, even though they're technically back muscles. Again: everything is connected.

There are many sources of upper back pain, including shoulder blades that have drifted too far apart. This is usually due to poor alignment along the thoracic vertebrae, a critical part of our Stack. When our chest muscles become too tight—often due to bad habits and imbalanced exercise choices—our shoulders round forward, which over stretches the upper back. Working with our arms in front of us for long periods of time can also cause this postural breakdown. Believe it or not, ignoring the Triangles beneath your feet can result in tightness high above the feet: in the thoracic spine. Without a strong, level foundation, the chest muscles can shorten and the shoulders can round forward, followed by the head. Such compensations are subtle and quiet, yet tenacious. Go back to the wall and see if your upper back and head rest comfortably against it. Unlike many structures in the body, the thoracic spine can actually find relief on the wall by allowing the muscles there to return to their preferred length instead of being constantly over-stretched. For some people, lying flat on the floor, with arms out to the sides and neck relaxed, will accomplish this as well. This combination of stretching tight chest muscles, relaxing overextended upper back muscles, and strengthening the muscles that retract the shoulder blades is a must for overall shoulder stability.

Moving our attention upward from the floor, our seven cervical vertebrae come next. These bones form the neck, a part of the spine that must be flexible enough to move our head into thousands of positions, yet sturdy enough to support the skull and everything inside it. (The human head can weigh as much as 12 pounds and the neck is its only means of support). Learning how to hold the head erect will develop and sustain the neck's proper curvature.

The cervical spine is where the canal for the spinal cord begins. It houses arteries that feed the base of the brain. Therefore, keeping the neck muscles strong and elastic is a must. For early hominids, a flexible cervical spine was a lifesaver! Our ancestors needed to turn their eyes, ears, and noses in all directions to stay aware of predators. For our Stacking purposes, though, maintaining proper posture and a level chin is good enough.

The neck can be challenged with all kinds of imbalances because of the many muscle groups involved in its function—not to mention the head it has to carry around. Typically, persons with a tight thoracic spine (upper back) carry their heads in front of their shoulders. The solution is to return the head and shoulders back to neutral. Return to your wall. Can you rest the back of your head comfortably against the wall while maintaining a level jawline? What if you try it while lying on your back? If you cannot accomplish this without tilting your chin up (away from your chest), then it's only a matter of time before your cervical spine will experience instability, pain, or injury.

Due to the large number of clients with this issue, we created a process that combines stretching the involved muscles (chest, traps, anterior shoulders, and the anterior and posterior thoracic musculature) with strengthening them. It is a slow process that cannot be rushed.

As your starting point, lie on your back with your knees bent and feet flat on the floor.

Place a cushion behind your head—one that will allow your neck to relax. Slowly spread your arms out to the side, palms facing up. From this position, slowly turn your head to the right while staying relaxed and breathing normally. Hold for 30 to 60 seconds. Repeat on the left side. As this becomes easier, reduce the size of the cushion behind your neck. Add arm movements, such as a weightless shoulder press. With the backs of your hands gliding across the floor, move your hands as if you are lifting two dumbbells over your head.

These movements start the process of releasing the hold that tight muscles have on the neck. Reduce the size of the support behind your head until you're lying flat on the floor with your neck comfortably in neutral. It's not unusual to work with the same size neck support for a few weeks. When you feel you've made sufficient progress on the floor, move to the wall.

Now would be a good time to return to our vision of building a Stack with alternating mobilizers and stabilizers. Remember this?

Mobilizer.

Stabilizer.

Mobilizer.

Stabilizer.

We were introduced to this idea through continued education and have found that it helps people who have lost connection the different muscle groups that encase our skeletons. We always start with the bottoms of the feet (stabilizers), then the ankles (mobilizers), moving up to the knees (stabilizers) and hip girdle (mobilizer). When we reach the spine, each intervertebral joint both mobilizes and stabilizes. Further proof that our backbones are truly a work of genius.

As we lift our focus to the shoulder girdle and arms, the importance of the chest and upper back will become clear. Once again, the wall stance will show us the way.

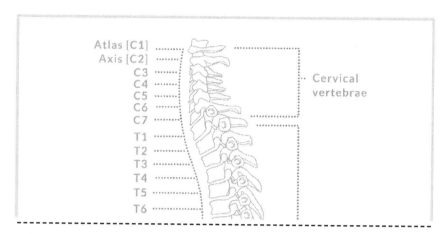

"It is not the strongest of the species that survives, nor the most intelligent that survives. It is the one that is the most adaptable to change."

- CHARLES DARWIN

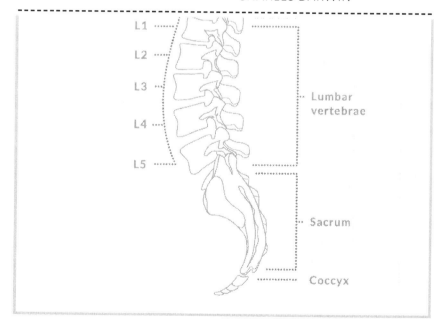

CHAPTER 6
Finding Your Core

THE RECTUS ABDOMINIS is the sheath of washboard-looking muscle that runs down the center of your torso, from the middle of the ribs to the pelvis. Behind it stands the transversus abdominis, the deepest muscle group in your core, which performs the crucial job of stabilizing your lumbar spine (low back). On each side of your torso is a set of oblique muscles, which are arranged at opposing angles in order to (1) aid rotation and (2) stabilize the torso over the hip girdle. Think of all these muscles as duct tape wrapped around the union of your upper and lower body, bound tightly to make sure your Stack doesn't slip.

The core involves other muscles as well, including:

» erector spinae on the lower spine

» the lower regions of the latissimus dorsi (the largest muscles of the back)

» smaller abdominal muscles like the pyramidalis

These miraculous muscles are rarely exercised, which makes little sense in that they comprise the most important muscle co-operative in our bodies.

There are muscle groups on the anterior (front) and posterior (back) of your torso whose only job is to balance your upper body over the center of the hips. Think about all the activity going on above the ribs: the movements of your shoulders, arms, chest, neck—and of course that valuable coconut at the top of it all. How does the torso stay stable and mobile? How can it swing a baseball bat 150 miles an hour and hold a motionless plank for minutes at a time?

As amazing as our core is, weak, tight muscles are its Kryptonite. People with sedentary lifestyles, or whose physical activities do not involve this part of the body, leave their core groups vulnerable. Here once again—the wall can expose weakness, especially in the transversus abdominis.

Many clients through the years have had such weaknesses exposed. Over time, we have noticed that there are similarities in their pain. Identifying these similarities allowed us to address the source.

Here are two examples how the body negatively adapts to weakness caused by lifestyle:

In the first example, a client complained of persistent lower back pain and tightness. We positioned the client against the wall, and immediately noticed too much extension in the lower spine—too much arch. The wall also revealed that the client had tight chest muscles and misplaced shoulders that kept the back of his head from touching the wall. After a complete assessment, the first step was to teach him where his hip hinge was. In doing this, it became clear that his lower back muscles, the ones that connect the upper body to the pelvic girdle, were overburdened. His shoulders were in front of his hips and he lacked strength and range of motion at the hip hinge. (Think of your waist as your beltline. Your hip hinge is below that, closer to your hip flexors.) His habit of bending at the waist and not the hinge kept his torso from sitting on its intended home. In short, he was using muscles that were not intended to support the weight of the torso.

His posture revealed other compensations due to his weak lumbar muscles and shortened rectus abdominis. He lacked a level foundation due to the supination (outward roll) of his foot, which added to the strain on his lower back. Your feet and your core may seem far apart, but they're a lot more connected than you think!

The second example also involved a client complaining of low back pain. In his case, the wall exposed a flat lower spine, with practically no arch. The chest muscles were so tight that his upper back and head could not properly make contact with the wall. As a result, his shoulder strength and range of motion were limited. Furthermore, his hips were tilted forward instead of staying in neutral. He involuntarily locked his knees when standing.

(Friendly reminder: the Wall is an amazing diagnostic tool! They are free and they are everywhere! In these two instances, the wall revealed hazardous compensations due to weak core muscles.)

These clients' lifestyles were different—one rarely exercised, the other exercised frequently, but with unstable posture. Our strategy for returning them to neutral was the same. We sought to activate the core while learning to stretch (release) the client's tight muscles.

We chose movements that released the anterior shoulder muscles and opened the chest. (This included stretching the biceps tendons at the top of the humerus.) We performed simple, safe neck stretches. We added exercises to stabilize his feet. Our hardest task—and our most time-consuming—was restoring full range of motion in the hip girdle. We employed various balance exercises, which not only activated his core muscles but strengthened his feet (Triangles). The combination of all this returned his torso to the home position: directly over the hips. Plus, he now had the strength and awareness to keep it there.

Every individual progresses at different speeds. Each of us responds differently to the same exercise. Be patient. Proceed according to your body's schedule, not one that your uninformed brain has invented.

Periodically remind yourself to work "from the bones out" instead of from the surface muscles in. Think about it: which is more important to proper movement, your bones or your skin? The answer is obvious, so keep your focus beneath what is visible with the naked eye.

The first step should always be to create stability. (What is stability? Envision yourself standing still in a tropical windstorm. That's stability. And it doesn't occur because your "mirror muscles" look pretty. It happens because your deepest muscles are properly aligned and doing their jobs.) Learning the difference between muscle activation and muscle tension is an important part of creating stability. Activating your deep postural muscles, mindfully and with focus, is the best way to stand your ground in that windstorm. Tense muscles create imbalance and distress.

To feel this for yourself, sit on a stability ball or the edge of a chair. You want the hip hinge to be neutral—at a clean, 90-degree angle—with your thighs aimed straight ahead and torso sitting straight up. Relax your shoulders and arms. Try and create a soft, neutral arch in your lumbar spine (low back). Lastly, activate your abdominal muscles—don't tense them!—gently pulling your abdominal wall closer to your spine. Think of your navel sinking into your torso without altering the shape of the spine.

Practice this same activation in different positions: lying on your back, standing against the Wall...

If you're feeling confident, do it while kneeling, or in a relaxed lunge position, focusing on your torso, not your legs. Now try it while in motion. If you feel lost or disconnected, drop into a "beginner's plank," a great way to remind yourself of the center of your body. Start by placing your forearms on an elevated surface such as a bench, then position your lower body in a pushup position, so that your body weight is shared by your forearms and toes (at the toe-joint line). Keep your torso activated, but not tense.

When you're feeling stronger, move away from the bench and place your forearms on the floor, joining your toes there so that your spine and the floor run parallel. The goal is to create a straight line from the top of your scalp, to your ankle joints, with a gentle arch in your low back. It's the same idea as the Wall Stance, except you're resisting gravity from a different angle. As your plank improves, focus on achieving the position without any tension in your body. We are seeking activation of your core muscles, not panic, strain, or stiffness.

If you feel your shoulders and arms becoming unstable before your core does, don't worry. Those muscles are the focus of our next chapter.

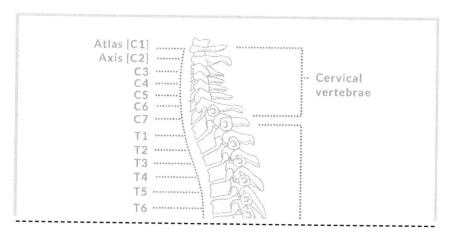

"He is able who thinks he is able!"

- CHINESE PROVERB

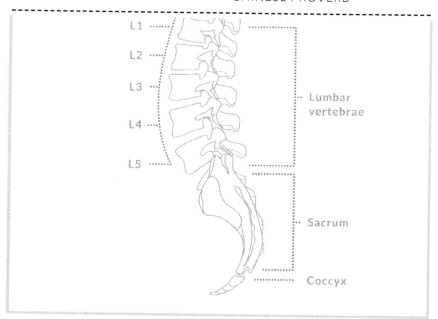

CHAPTER 7
Shoulder Girdle and Arms

ANTHROPOLOGICALLY, one of the most compelling differences between hominids and other mammals is our dexterity. Not just with our most distant appendages, our fingers, but with the powerful, precise machines known as shoulders and arms.

The shoulder girdle, also referred to as the pectoral girdle, is formed by the clavicles and the shoulder blades (scapulae). If you were to look down on the top of your head, these four bones would form a diamond shape, with your head at the center of the diamond. The two most distant points on the diamond are the shoulder joints, the points of attachment for the upper arm—the sockets into which the humerus bone inserts. The humerus is kept in that socket by muscles that connect it to the axial skeleton (the central part of your skeleton: ribs, sternum, spine). The shoulder joint, in fact, represents our strongest connection between the sternum (in front) and the spinal column (in back).

Sounds fairly simple with such a small number of bones involved, but don't be fooled. There are also the elbow, lower arm, wrist, and hand to consider, as well as the cervical spine and head; and we need to put all of this in motion, too, of course. Is it any wonder why our shoulders carry such a disproportionate amount of the stress and tension in our bodies?

When you think about the shoulders and arms in terms of their workload (which is also disproportionately large) and in terms of their ranges of motion and infinite movement possibilities, they rank among the most complicated and vulnerable parts of our entire musculoskeletal system. In other words, they're amazing, but lots can go wrong.

When helping individuals become more in tune with their body, the shoulder is always one of the most challenging areas to address. The ability to maintain evenly balanced strength in the shoulder joint requires an understanding of where that strength originates. Not only for exercise or sport, but our daily activities. (Mothers of small children, this shoulder massage goes out to you!)

Hopefully we have demonstrated so far in this book that each group of bones and muscles depends on those above and below it. The hip girdle counts on there being a level foundation at the feet. The torso and spine depend on a level hip girdle. The shoulders rely directly on the spine. When there's an issue with any of these relationships, the neck and head are often left vulnerable, especially when there is poor shoulder alignment. In this area, as with others, constructing our Stack requires a combination of flexibility and strength.

As always, we'll focus first on the deepest muscles—the ones that connect the bones to their innermost joint. In the shoulder, that's a group of four muscles referred to as the rotator cuff. The rotator cuff surrounds the head of the humerus (the long bone in the upper arm) and is anchored to the scapulae. The dictionary, by the way, defines cuff as "a small sleeve," and that's precisely what this is. This small sleeve confines the mobility of our arms within a safe range of motion. Think of all the things our arms can do: throw, press, punch, pull, lift, reach, hold a squirming toddler. Each of these movements requires the development of muscles that stabilize our scapulae.

We won't turn this into an anatomy lesson, but there is a lot of confusion out there about how the shoulder functions. Knowing how many muscles and bones are involved—if not memorizing their names—helps us understand each part's importance. The shoulder is definitely a brick within your Stack that needs to be aligned and in control before quality arm movement can begin. That said, the number of people who have come to us with no knowledge of what they did to cause their shoulder issues is alarming. As with the back, most came to us seeking relief from shoulder pain or limited range of motion. The percentage of people who have come to us with known structural issues—a diagnosed ligament tear or strained rotator cuff—is small by comparison.

As with Debbie's scoliosis, some individuals are born with irregular bone shapes. Although the bones are off their natural alignment, they still have muscles attached to them—muscles that these people need for their everyday lives, muscles that require extra attention because of the nearby bone irregularity.

When the scapulae is retracted and stable—not floating around or hunching forward—the shoulders and arms have a safe anchor from which to move. The largest percentage of shoulder injuries results from poor scapula position during arm movement. Even those of us who are in "great shape" fail to realize the need for balance between the large back muscles and large chest muscles.

Quick story:

Back when we were first learning to train with weights in the mid-70s—when heavier always meant better—we had a friend who would do chest and shoulders three days a week. He was strong. He benched 450 pounds for one rep. He squatted 350 and shoulder pressed an impressive 225. But he never trained his back muscles. One day Norm asked him why.

"I get enough back work doing squats," he replied. "And besides, why work on what you can't see? Hahahahaha."

Thirty years later he had the first of two shoulder replacements. We're convinced that his choice to ignore his latissimus dorsi muscles—critical stabilizers of the posterior shoulder—played a significant role in his need for artificial shoulder joints. You can hardly blame the guy no one knew better back then. Today, this need for balanced training is pretty common knowledge. Unfortunately, this old 1970s "chest and arms" routine is still widely practiced. Ignore your posterior half at your own peril, Stackers!

There is a reason for every muscle in our body. Every one of them has an assignment. Usually several assignments. If these muscles are prevented from doing their jobs for some reason, their workload has to be picked up by another muscle, which may or may not be prepared for it. Our bodies aren't put into motion by a single muscle, but rather by groups of muscles. The smaller the number of muscles involved, the greater the chance of imbalanced workload and compensation.

Stacking, in essence, means building your posture with balanced strength within the different planes of the body: front, back, left, right, top, bottom. When this is accomplished, we can keep our bones in their pockets, preventing unnecessary injuries and premature wear and tear. As we like to put it: Where there's a muscle there's a reason.

When we assess a client experiencing shoulder discomfort, finding the culprit is rarely a problem. (Many times, we've been able to reveal an imbalance before pain has surfaced, just by looking at the feet during a Wall Stance.) The main issue is determining how much damage has already been done. We always tell our clients to get a medical diagnosis first, to determine if any surgical repair is needed. If surgery cannot be avoided, physical therapy, along with our Stacking training, needs to take place or the injury will most likely return.

Our best rule of thumb for shoulder health is this: a well-positioned shoulder blade—gently retracted, never shrugged upward or rounded forward—is the foundation for quality arm movement. The reason is because, as we stated earlier, the scapulae anchor the rotator cuff.

Well-positioned scapulae also allow the large muscles on the front and back of the torso (including the pectoralis and latissimus) to stabilize the area. And they allow smaller muscles, with odd names like teres major and coracobrachialis, to help these larger muscles provide movement.

In addition to these stabilizers and movers there is the deltoid, the main shoulder muscle visible just under the skin. The "delt" offers a great example of how a large, primary mover is dependent on the smaller muscles surrounding it. Our bodies crave balance. We have been given the muscles to achieve that goal. The trick is to use them as they were intended.

Are you old enough to remember all those cases of carpal tunnel syndrome back in the 80s? At the time, the popularity of personal computers received the blame. Today, stress on the thumbs brought on by texting has become an issue. Because our hands are so far removed from our Stack, they don't require as much attention as, say, our knees and shoulders, in terms of injury prevention, but they do require some attention.

Where the fingers are concerned, our device-dependent lifestyles can shorten our flexors (which curl the fingers) and weaken our extensors (which straighten them). When we assess clients, we don't stop when our postural tests are done. Common arm and hand issues we see include: (1) elbows that do not completely straighten when hanging at the sides, (2) tight wrist extensors that pull the back of the hand toward the forearm, and (3) fingers that overcurl into the palm when relaxed.

Next time life hands you a five-minute break, don't check your phone. Stretch your wrists and fingers. You don't have to know the name of each muscle, or memorize its function, but this often-ignored part of your body deserves at least a little bit of love.

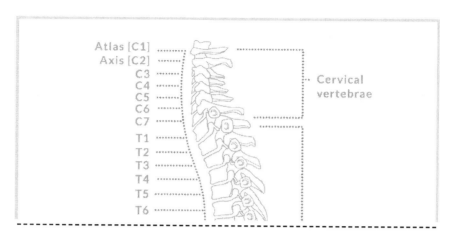

"Tell me and I forget, teach me and I remember, involve me and I learn."

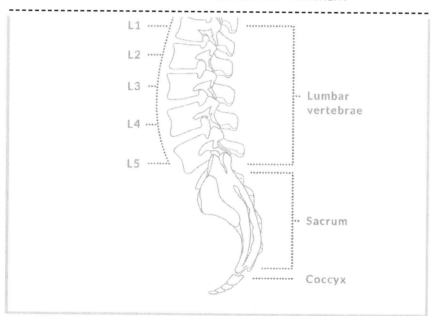

CHAPTER 8
Neck and Head

CONGRATULATIONS. We're almost finished stacking our skeleton. Think about all we've learned so far: from the level foundation of our Triangles, to the long bones that rise from them to form our legs, to the intricate lattice-work of our pelvis and spine, plus the muscles and other soft tissues that glue this whole complex system together.

And it's all there for one purpose: to safely cradle your cranium as you put your body in motion. If your Stack is properly built at every level beneath your shoulders, but has a brick out of place at neck-level, pain will result, and over time, your skyscraper of a body might even start to lean. So let's finish strong.

Your head weighs about 11 pounds. That's roughly eight percent of your total body mass, so it isn't as light as it seems. Muscle control is important here. This doesn't mean tension. You shouldn't have to force your head into its proper place. What we're seeking is something we call "flexible activation," which allows movement in virtually any direction while safeguarding the cervical spine. Flexible activation keeps the bones of your neck in their respective pockets. It can take time to learn, so don't get discouraged. Just trust the process. Think: activation without tension.

A productive starting point is to imagine a thread attached to the top of your head that gently lifts your scalp toward the sky. This thin thread doesn't yank your head upward. There's no straining. Threads snap when yanked or strained. It just lifts, while allowing you to maintain a level jaw line.

The most common imbalance at this level appears in those whose heads rest in front of their shoulders. There are many causes for this, including daily driving, cell phone use, and computer use. (One hidden influence can be the size of your pillow. We have worked with clients whose necks were being wrenched sideways six to eight hours each day during sleep. Talk about a silent killer! If your Stack improves but you're still experiencing neck pain or headaches, consider asking a medical specialist about your pillow.) All of these things can cause bad postural habits, and over time, they add up.

The lesson here is: the further your head is in front of your shoulders, the harder it is to place your head against the wall during the Wall Stance. It's a common issue, so don't feel bad if you're out of whack in this area.

Although this is our last group of bones and muscles, with nothing above them that depends on them, the weight of the head and the curvature of the neck requires the jaw position to be level. Dessert makers don't place a cherry on the side of a sundae. It goes on top.

In the two chapters titled The Wall, and Spine, the shape of the cervical vertebrae and placement of head were discussed. As with every section of our Stack, visualizing the bones and muscles involved makes it easier to make adjustments when needed. We have several deep muscles in our necks that control the throat and the stacking of our cervical vertebrae. The ones we're most concerned with are the larger, superficial muscles that control the cervical spine and head. We're simplifying a bit, but it suffices to say: the neck and its connection to the head is a complicated structure.

Moving the head and positioning it on top of the cervical spine is the responsibility of two large muscles. There's the long, vertical muscle on each side of the throat called the sternocleidomastoid, which originates from the collarbone and connects right behind each ear. And in the back, there's the trapezius, the thick, trapezoid-shaped muscles that originate at the thoracic vertebrae and end at the posterior base of the skull. (The "traps" also support the scapulae and move the arms.)

Both of these muscles—the sternocleidomastoid and trapezius—control the rotation, extension, and flexion of the skull. They are constantly in control of the head, in all of its positions, at every angle, either together or individually. These muscles are in their preferred, neutral state when the lower jaw line is parallel with the floor and the ears are over the shoulders.

The shape of the neck and the position of the head are two of the biggest factors in creating proper posture. They are also the final two factors in building our Stacks from the ground up. That thin, imaginary thread at the top of your scalp, after all, is nothing more than a silky extension of your Stack, which is constructed of durable, mineral-infused bone. Your skeleton works in levers and cantilevers, balls and sockets, backbones and intervertebral discs. If we've Stacked it correctly, it is as stable at the top as it is on the soles of your feet. Now it's time to move.

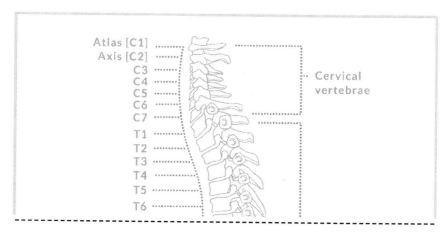

"What would life be if we had no courage to attempt anything?"

- VINCENT VAN GOGH

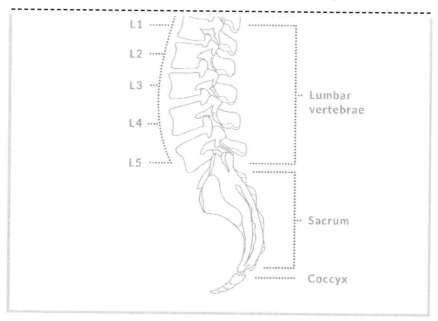

CHAPTER 9
Posture in Motion

HOPEFULLY BY NOW you can see that our musculoskeletal systems aren't just 206 bones with a bunch of ligaments, tendons, and muscles tossed onto the heap. Each of us is a miracle of structural engineering. We hope also that this book has pointed out the need for communication between these structures, a requirement for keeping our bones in their pockets.

Our concept of Stacking was born from our clients' needs, and our own battles with scoliosis (Debbie) and repeated traumatic injury and recovery (Norm). Initially, we saw that our Stacks contained three different foundations, at the (1) feet, (2) hips, and (3) shoulders. We envisioned these as three flat plateaus on the side of a mountain—stable places upon which we can continue to build the structures above. This approach also helped us rethink the way we can bring a body back from injury. They say that necessity is the mother of invention, and that's certainly true in our case. Necessity forced us to invent something that could make sense to anyone, something that had also been tested and proven by our own experiences. Because of the time we've spent with clients who had serious issues like spina bifida, Parkinson's, fibromyalgia, club foot, fused vertebrae, and joint replacements, we were able to create an assessment process that soon became invaluable to everyone on our client list. Stacking has become part of our clients' lives, and the benefits have been remarkable for us to witness—particularly when the Stacks we've helped build are put it into motion.

Dozens of friends and clients have come to us thinking they knew what they needed, only to find themselves stunned by what our assessment exposed. This is why we start everyone off with the same assessments. Everyone's Stack is different, but the steps for building your best Stack are the same for all.

The wall will be your best tool. Look first to expose weaknesses in the foundation, then address them as you move upward, progressing, looking for imbalances as well as bones that aren't resting in their pockets. It starts the moment you get out of bed. When your bones are correctly placed and aimed in the right direction it allows the ligaments, tendons, and muscles to be at their correct length and their strongest position for the remainder of the day ... for the remainder of your life.

Try and find your Pain Free Zone, without compensating. From this neutral position we're able to find our greatest strength. Remember: when you're strong in neutral, you're strong everywhere.

Our Stacks are capable of doing amazing things as we age. Look at Ella Mae Colbert, 100 years young, who recently broke the world record for the 100-yard dash in her age group. You may not be interested in becoming a world record sprinter at age 100. The point is, when our skeletal structures are in their proper places, aging becomes easier and restrictive pain is reduced.

When we learn to delegate work to the correct muscle groups, we change bad habits into good habits. When you learn that a balanced Triangle is your foundation, that the Wall is the perfect tool to reset your Stack, then you will always have a place—anywhere you go—where you can check in and realign. Try it out before your next big business meeting (or world-record sprint attempt!).

When you learn that the hip girdle is your center of gravity and your shoulder girdle is the anchor for your neck and head, you'll have a body that is settled and aware. With practice, you'll have muscles that will know how to bring their bones back to neutral.

Our bones, after all, only go where our muscles take them.

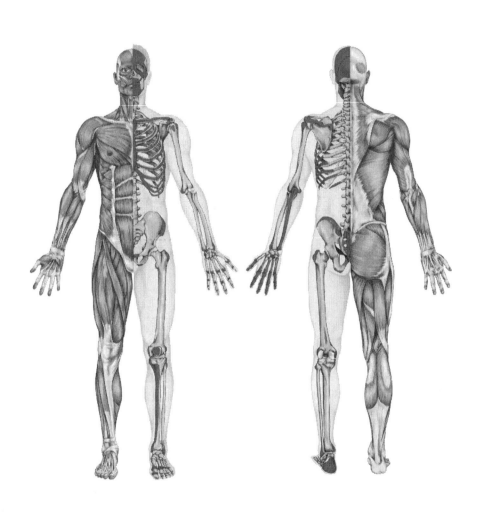

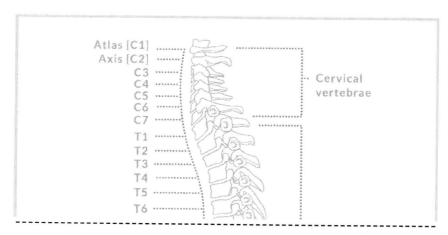

"Live your life on purpose."

- WAYNE DYER

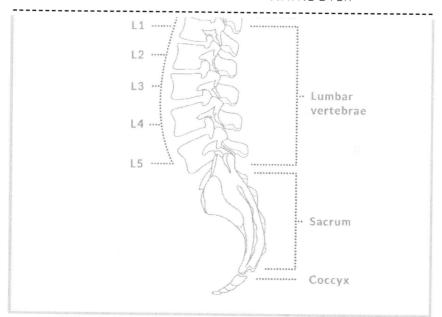

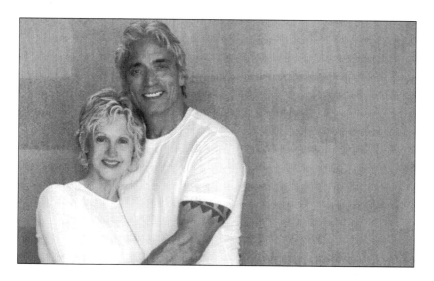

DEB AND NORM have been married for 38 years and have been physically active since they met in 1976. They began their connection to the fitness world through a variety of certifications and continuing education programs such as Health Coach and Medical Exercise Specialist. In addition to being an athlete his whole life, Norm was a Hollywood stuntman for 27 years. The combination of personal challenges and the variety of clients who have crossed their paths have comprised the most important part of Norm and Deb's education.

Made in the USA
San Bernardino, CA
25 June 2017